ULTRA-PROCESSED FOODS

The untold story…….

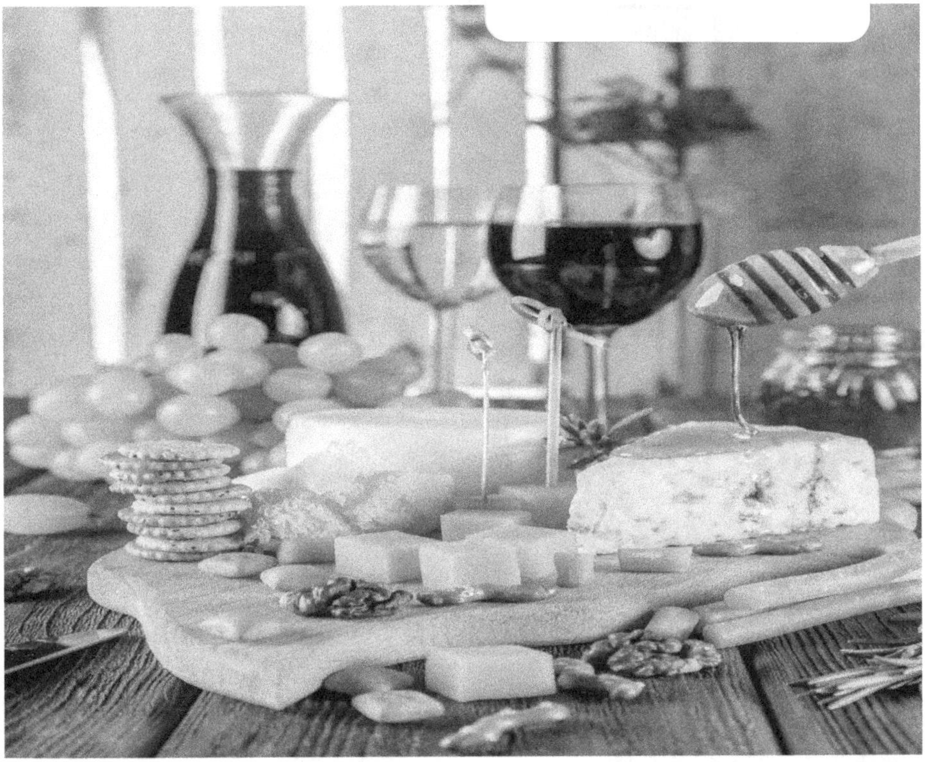

SUCCESS T. HELEN

Table of Content

__INTRODUCTION__

__Chapter 1__

__Foods and Processed Food__

__Chapter 2__

__Historical Context and Evolution of Ultra-processed foods__

__Chapter 3__

__Nutritional Composition of Ultra-processed Foods__

__Chapter 4__

__The Impact of Ultra-processed Foods on Human Health__

__Chapter 5__

__Socioeconomic and Environmental Consequences__

__Chapter 6__

__Consumer Behavior and Food Choices__

__Chapter 7__

__Regulatory Framework and Policy Responses__

__Chapter 8__

__Alternatives and Solutions for Ultra-processed Foods__

__Chapter 9__

__Case Studies and Success Stories__

__Chapter 10__

__Future Perspectives and Recommendations__

__Conclusion__

INTRODUCTION

Ultra-processed foods now account for two-thirds of calories in diets worldwide. If more than 20% of your daily calorie consumption includes ultra-processed foods, you may be upping your risk for health deterioration. However, many of our basic foods, such as wheat, dairy, refined sugars, and oils were introduced during the agricultural and industrial revolutions. They have substituted a better pre-agricultural revolution diet that comprised nutrition-packed lean meats, fish, and fresh fruits and vegetables. As a result, many contemporary individuals have yet to experience the delight of clean eating.

One simple technique to ensure diet quality is to cook and prepare your meals from scratch.

"We claim we don't have time, yet it doesn't take that much time.

It is crucial to recognize from the beginning that no fitness goal can be attained without eating clean. A healthy diet is key to optimum health. If you consume trash, you attract illnesses.

On the other hand nutritious, whole, and fresh food is your passport to life, greater health, and long life.

Chapter 1

Foods and Processed Food

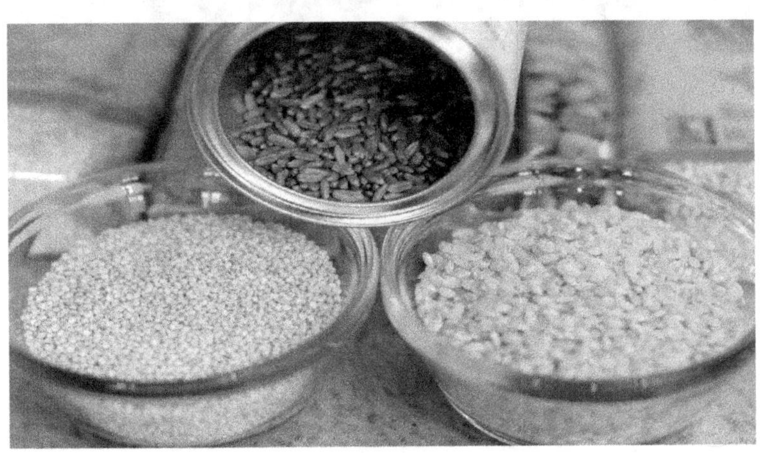

Food is typically described as any material taken by an organism for nutritional support. Food is generally of plant, animal, or fungal origin, and provides important elements, such as carbs, lipids, proteins, vitamins, or minerals. The material is taken by an organism and absorbed by the organism's cells to supply energy, sustain life, or encourage growth.

It is typically suggested to "eat less processed food."

Classification of foods based on the processing

1) Unprocessed or natural: Foods that originate straight from plants or animals and aren't changed at all.

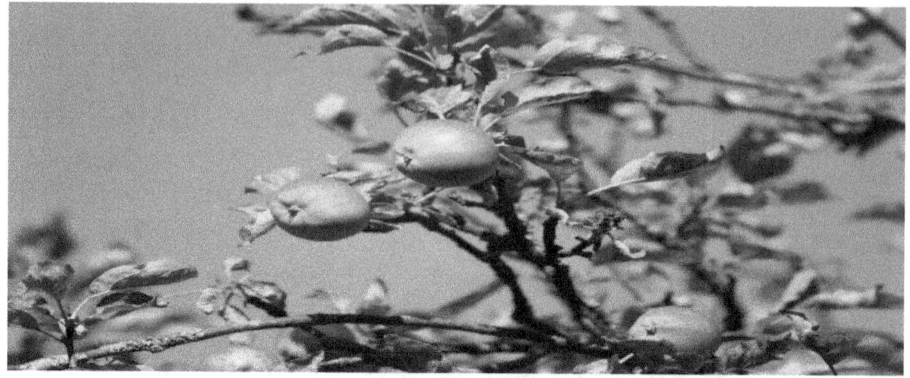

2) Minimally processed foods: are entire foods in which the vitamins and minerals are still intact. The food is in its natural (or almost natural) condition. These foods may be slightly changed by removal of inedible components, drying, crushing, roasting, boiling, freezing, or pasteurization, to make them appropriate to store and safe to ingest. Unprocessed or little processed foods would include carrots, apples, raw poultry, melon, and raw, unsalted almonds.

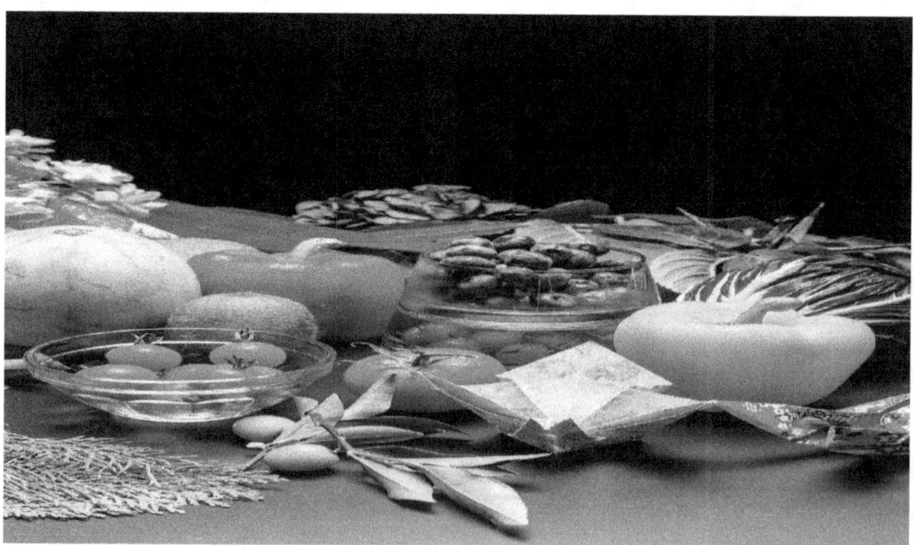

3) Processed transformed foods:

Processed foods are generally manufactured by adding salt, oil, sugar, or other things - but are derived from natural or lightly processed foods and identifiable as these foods. Examples include canned fish or canned veggies, fruits in syrup, and freshly prepared bread. Most processed foods include two or three components.

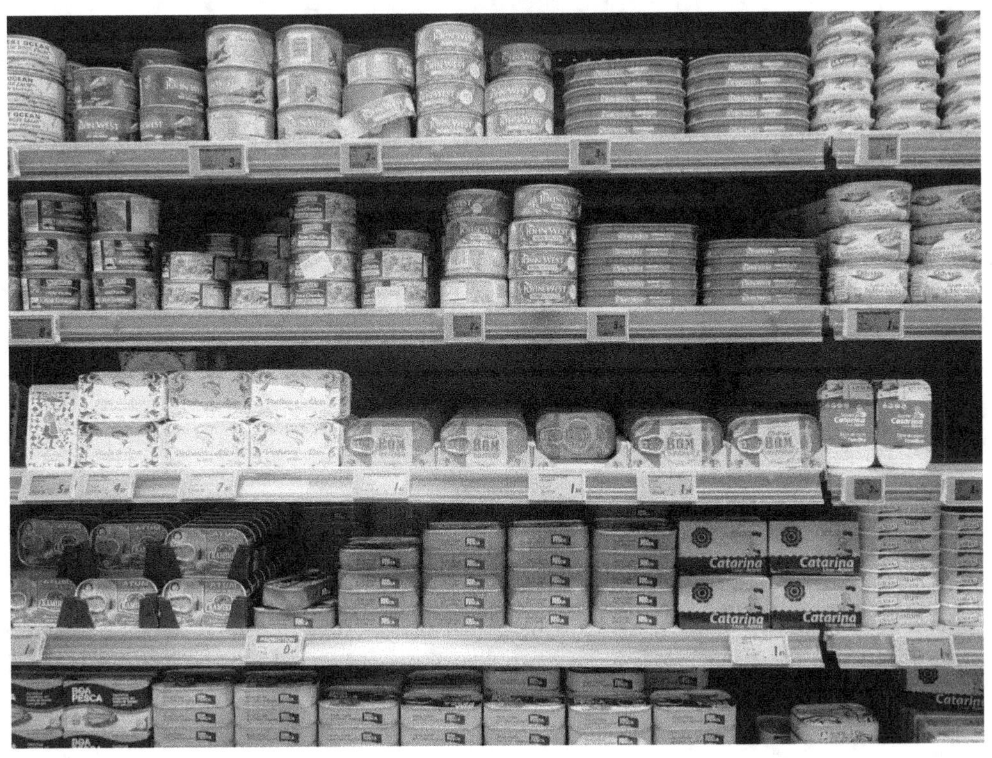

4) Extremely processed foods or ultra-processed: Industrially manufactured foods contain practically full compounds taken from foods like oils, fats, sugars, starches, and proteins, or created in laboratories and factories with few, if any, elements that originate directly from natural plants or animal sources.

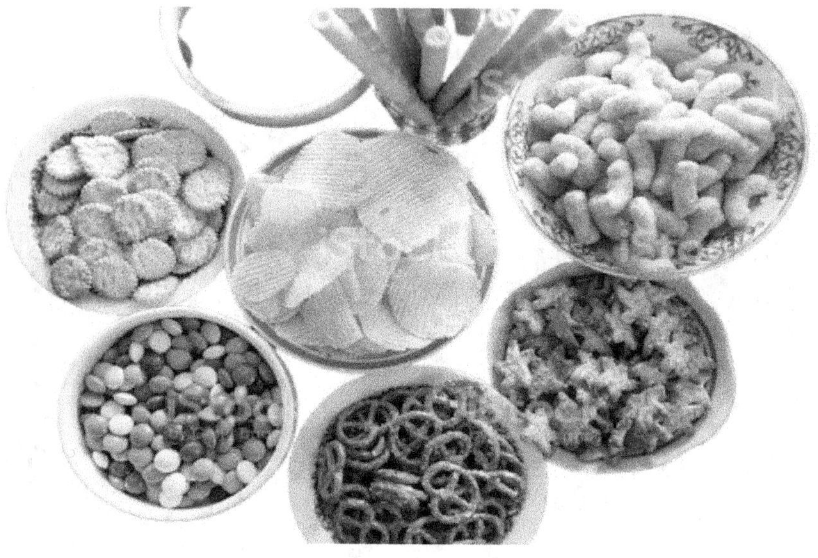

Examples of ultra-processed meals

Ultra-processed foods are highly processed and generally include a mixture of multiple components, including added sugars, fats, and preservatives. They are frequently intended to be handy, shelf-stable, and attractive to the customer. Some examples of ultra-processed foods include:

- Packaged snack items such as chips, crackers, and cookies
- Frozen dinners and pizza
- Soft drinks and other sugary beverages
- Processed meats such as hot dogs, bacon, and deli meats
- Packaged baked items such as cakes, pastries, and doughnuts
- Instant noodles and soups
- Frozen dinners and microwaveable meals
- Flavored yogurts and dairy desserts
- Energy bars and sports drinks
- Instant oatmeal and breakfast cereals
- Packaged bread and rolls
- Candy and chocolate bars
- Processed cheese and cheese products
- Packaged sauces and condiments

Ultra-processed foods…….

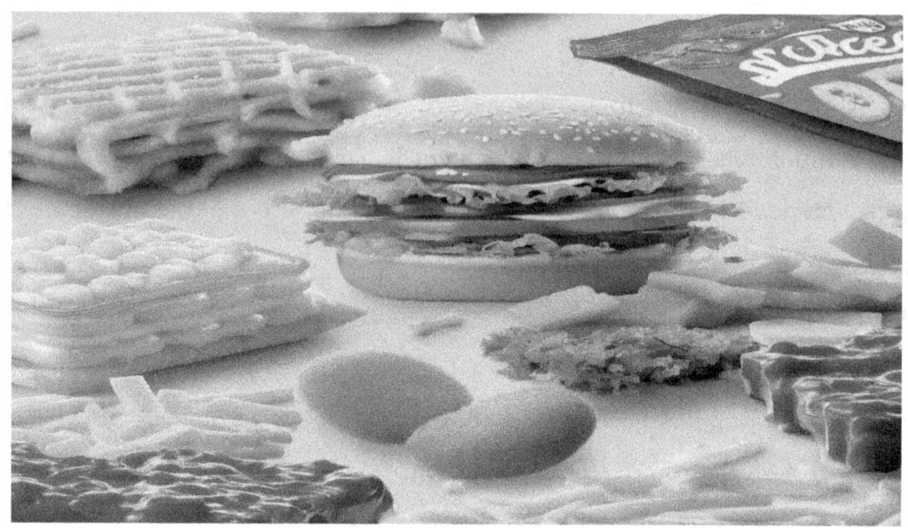

Chapter 2

Historical Context and Evolution of Ultra-processed foods

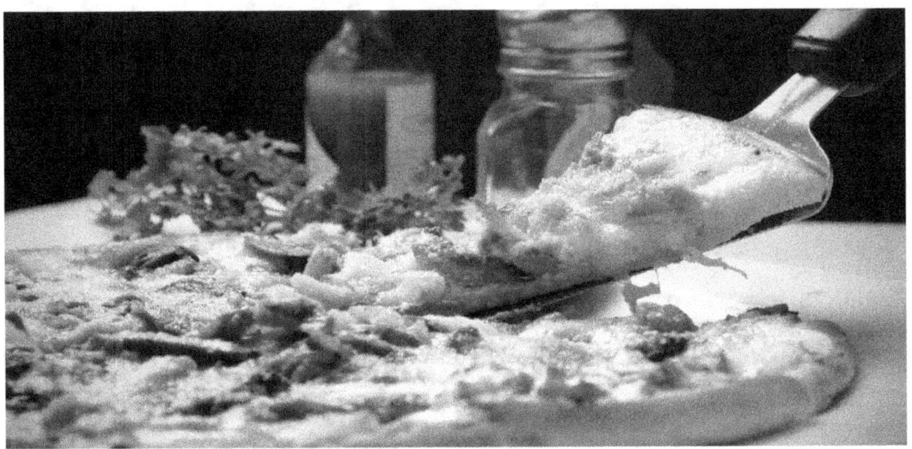

Take a fascinating journey to **explore** the historical roots and evolution of ultra-processed foods. It's like unlocking the secrets of our modern-day food landscape.

a) Ancient Beginnings: Our narrative begins thousands of years ago, when people first started growing crops and domesticating animals for nourishment. Food back then was simple, fresh mostly whole grains, fruits, vegetables, lean meats, and minimally processed natural foods.

b) Industrial Revolution: The Industrial Revolution changed how food was produced and consumed in the 18th and 19th centuries. Advances in technology brought in the mass production of food with the invention of machinery for milling grains, canning fruits and vegetables, and refining sugar. This marked the beginning of widespread food processing on an industrial scale.

c) Early Innovations: As the 20th century got underway, food processing was developing rapidly. The food industry was completely transformed by inventions such as pasteurization, refrigeration, and the development of chemical additives. These advances led to the creation of new, highly processed food items in addition to extending the shelf life of foods.

d) Post-War **Boom:** Food processing and manufacturing experienced a boom in the years after World War II, driven by factors such as rising demand, advances in technology, and changing consumer preferences. As convenience became a top priority, ready-to-eat meals, packaged snacks, and other highly processed foods meant for rapid and simple consumption became more popular.

e) Globalization and Commoditization: As the world became more interconnected, food production and distribution became increasingly globalized. Consequently, food became more and more of a commodity, with multinational companies controlling the market and driving the global acceptance of ultra-processed meals.

f) The Era of Digital Technology: As we fast-forward to the present, we discover that we live in the digital era, where technology continues to shape our food system in unprecedented ways. The convenience of highly processed meals is now more widely accessible than ever before via the development of online grocery shopping and food delivery apps.

g) Looking Ahead: As we analyze the historical background and evolutionary history of ultra-processed foods, it is important to take into account their effects on our health, the environment, and society at large. These foods are convenient and affordable, but they pose significant challenges in terms of food security, sustainability, and nutrition. Through comprehending their history and development, we may make knowledgeable decisions about the foods we consume

and work towards creating a more sustainable, healthful food future for future generations.

Essential Features of Ultra-processed Foods

<u>Ultra-processed</u> foods are a kind of food items that go through extensive industrial processing, involving multiple stages of chemical manipulation, refining, and adding different artificial ingredients. These foods are usually distinguished by their high level of processing, the absence of whole, natural ingredients, and their dependence on additives and refined materials.

Essential Features of Ultra-processed foods include:

1) Complexity of Ingredients: Ultraprocessed meals consist of a wide variety of components, many of which are not common in household kitchens. Common examples of these ingredients include refined sugars, hydrogenated oils, artificial coloring, flavorings, and preservatives. Other additives include thickeners, stabilizers, and emulsifiers.

2) Industrial Processing: These foods undergo a lot of industrial processing, which often includes chemical treatments, high pressure, and temperatures. Processing techniques include extrusion, milling, refining, and chemical manipulation which may remove natural nutrients and change the composition of the original materials.

3) Minimal Whole Foods: Ultra-processed foods contain minimal quantities of whole, natural nutrients including fruits, vegetables, whole grains, and lean proteins. Rather than this, they depend heavily on refined and processed products, which may not have the same nutritional benefits of dietary fiber as whole foods.

4) Highly Palatable: Ultra-processed foods, due to the formulation and processing methods used are often designed to be highly palatable, with intense flavors, textures, and mouthfeels. These characteristics may encourage overconsumption and contribute to the development of unhealthy eating habits.

5) Convenience and Shelf Stability: Ultra-processed foods are easily accessible and easy to eat because of their lengthy shelf life and simple design. However, their prolonged shelf stability often comes at the expense of nutritional quality, as they may contain high levels of added sugars, unhealthy fats, and sodium.

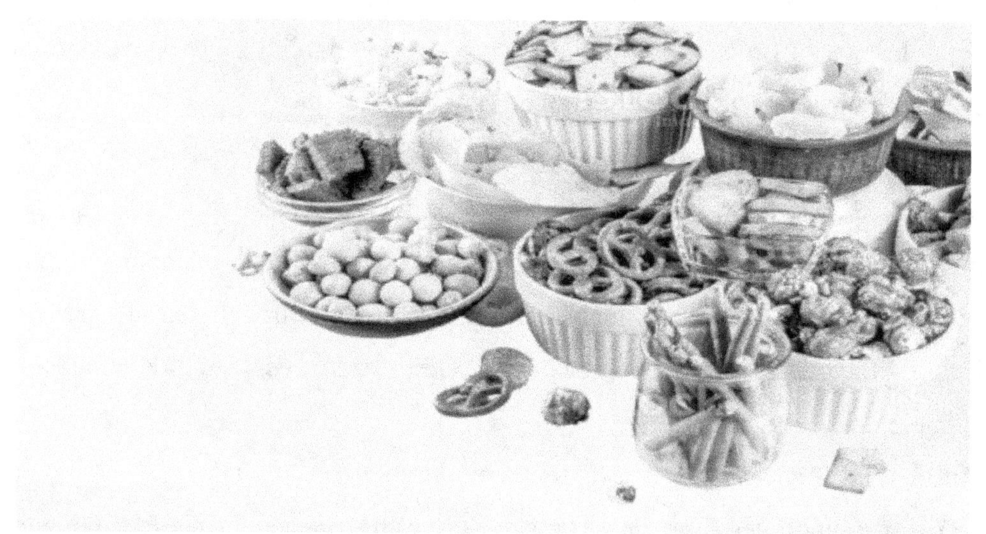

Factors Responsible for Global Trends and Consumption Patterns of Ultra-processed foods

The factors responsible for the global and consumption trends of intriguing Ultra-processed foods and how they are influencing the state of the food industry today are examined below:

1) Quick Development: The use of ultra-processed foods has increased significantly over the last few decades globally. This trend is driven by several factors which include urbanization, changing lifestyles, more disposable income, and the globalization of food markets. The market for ready-to-eat, quick meals has expanded as more people migrate into cities and embrace Westernized diets.

2) Urbanization and Westernisation: Urbanization plays a crucial role in driving the consumption of ultra-processed foods. As people migrate to cities in quest of better economic opportunities, they often adopt urban lifestyles which are characterized by rapid living, longer working hours, and less time for home cooking. This shift towards urbanization is accompanied by a transition to Westernized diets, which are typically high in ultra-processed foods, such as fast food, packaged snacks, and sugary beverages.

3) Globalization of Food Markets: One reason why ultraprocessed foods are so widely available and consumed is because of the globalization of food markets. Multinational food corporations have expanded their reach into new markets, bringing with them a wide range of ultra-processed products catered to local tastes and preferences.

As a result of globalization, food cultures have become more homogenized, and ultra-processed meals are now more prevalent in areas where they were formerly less prevalent.

4) Marketing and Advertising: The promotion of ultra-processed food consumption is mostly attributed to the marketing and promotional tactics used by food firms. Employing focused marketing initiatives, product placements, and celebrity endorsements, these businesses establish a powerful attraction around their offerings, compelling customers to buy and use them. Furthermore, ultra-processed foods' branding and packaging often communicate ideas of cost, prestige, and convenience, which contribute to their appeal.

5) The Role of Policy: Globally, governments and public health groups are increasingly realizing that policy actions are necessary to combat the use of ultra-processed foods. These might include measures like enforcing laws governing food labeling, restricting the marketing of unhealthy foods to children, implementing taxes on sugar-filled drinks, and promoting healthier food options in schools, workplaces, and communities.

Chapter 3

Nutritional Composition of Ultra-processed Foods

Macronutrient and Micronutrient Profiles

Here, let's delve into the intricate world of macro and micronutrients found in ultra-processed meals and learn more about the complicated makeup that makes these goods what they are.

Macronutrients:

1) Carbohydrates: Ultra-processed foods often contain high concentrations of refined carbohydrates, such as sugars and white flour. These carbs are absorbed fast in the bloodstream, which may cause a sharp rise in blood sugar levels and disruptions in insulin sensitivity. Furthermore, additional sugars are included in a lot of ultra-processed meals, which raises the product's calorie density and adds to its overall carbohydrate contents.

2) Fats: Many ultra-processed foods are high in unhealthy fats, such as trans fats and saturated fats, which are often added to enhance texture, flavor, and shelf stability.

When consumed in excess, these fats have been associated with some chronic and other metabolic problems. Moreover, ultra-processed meals contain hydrogenated oils, which include trans fats linked to negative health consequences.

3) Proteins: While meat, poultry, and dairy products are potential sources of protein in certain ultra-processed meals, many others depend on less costly protein sources

like soy protein isolate or textured vegetable protein. These protein sources could be enhanced nutritionally by additions, but they might not have the total amino acid profile seen in real meals.

Micronutrients:

1) Vitamins: Whole, unprocessed meals include critical vitamins and minerals that are often absent from ultraprocessed diets. The vitamins and minerals that are naturally contained in the raw materials may be removed by the refining and processing methods used to make these goods. While vitamins and minerals may be added to certain ultra-processed meals to fortify their nutritional content, the body may not absorb or utilize these additives as quickly as it would if the nutrients were present in whole foods.

2) Minerals: Likewise, foods that have undergone extreme processing (ultra-processed foods) could be deficient in vital minerals including calcium, magnesium, iron, and zinc. These minerals are essential for physiological functions such as the health of bones, muscle functions, and the immune system, among others. However, these minerals may be lost during the processing and refinement of components in ultra-processed meals, leading to potential nutrient deficiencies in individuals who rely heavily on these products for their diet.

3) Antioxidants and Phytonutrients: Antioxidants and phytonutrients are naturally occurring substances found in fruits, vegetables, and whole grains. Ultraprocessed diets typically contain minimal amounts of these nutrients. These substances help to protect the body against oxidative stress and inflammation and have been connected to a lower chance of developing chronic illnesses and neurological problems. Ultraprocessed foods' total nutritional value is decreased by the degradation or removal of these beneficial compounds caused by the processing and refining of their constituents.

ADDITIVES, PRESERVATIVES, AND FLAVOR ENHANCERS

It is necessary to explore the complicated world of flavor enhancers, preservatives, and additives found in ultraprocessed foods uncovering the wide range of substances that contribute to their texture, taste, and shelf stability.

A) ADDITIVES:

1) Artificial Colors: Artificial colors are often added to ultra-processed meals to improve their visual appeal and make them more attractive to customers. These colors are meant to mimic the natural hues of fruits, vegetables, and other ingredients and may be derived artificially.

2) Artificial Flavors: Manufacturers of ultra-processed meals often add artificial flavors made from synthetic chemicals to improve the food's taste and aroma. These flavors may be applied to a variety of products to produce certain flavor profiles since they are designed to mimic the taste of real foods like fruits, spices, and herbs.

3) Emulsifiers: Emulsifiers are substances applied to aid the blending together of materials that would not normally combine, such as water and oil, to enhance the texture and stability of ultra-processed foods. Emulsifiers that are commonly added to processed foods like margarine, mayonnaise, and salad dressings include lecithin, mono-and diglycerides, and polysorbates.

4) Stabilizers and Thickeners: Stabilultraprocessedizers and thickeners are additives used to enhance the mouthfeel, texture, and ultra-processed foods. These substances assist in preventing separation and aid in keeping the product's texture consistent throughout. Commonly used stabilizers and thickeners are carrageenan, guar gum, and xanthan gum which are commonly applied to processed foods such as ice cream, sauces, and soups.

B) PRESERVATIVES

1) Antioxidants: Antioxidants are preservatives employed in ultra-processed meals to prevent the oxidation of fats and oils, which may cause rancidity and unpleasant tastes. Tocopherols (vitamin E) and butylated hydroxytoluene (BHT), butylated hydroxyanisole (BHA) are common antioxidants that are added to processed foods such as snack bars, morning cereals, and fried meals to increase their shelf life.

2) Antimicrobial Agents: Antimicrobial agents are preservatives that are used in ultra-processed foods to prevent the development of bacteria, yeasts, and molds, prolonging their shelf life and lowering the risk of spoilage. Common antimicrobial agents are sorbic acid, benzoic acid, and propionic acid, and are added to processed foods such as cheese, bread, and processed meats.

C) Flavor Enhancers:

1) Monosodium Glutamate (MSG): MSG is a flavor enhancer that is often utilized to provide a savory or umami flavor to ultra-processed foods. It is derived from glutamic acid, an amino which is naturally present in several foods including cheese, mushrooms, and tomatoes. MSG is often added to improve the taste and palatability of these processed meals including soups, sauces, and snack foods.

2) Yeast Extracts: Yeast extracts are natural flavor enhancers made from yeast cells. They are used to improve the savory taste of ultra-processed meals. They have naturally occurring glutamic acid and additional flavorings which contribute to the umami taste. Yeast extracts are often added to enhance the taste and fragrance of processed foods like sauces, ready-to-eat meals, and savory snacks. Although regulatory agencies usually consider these compounds to be safe for ingestion, there have been concerns expressed about the possible health implications of excessive consumption.

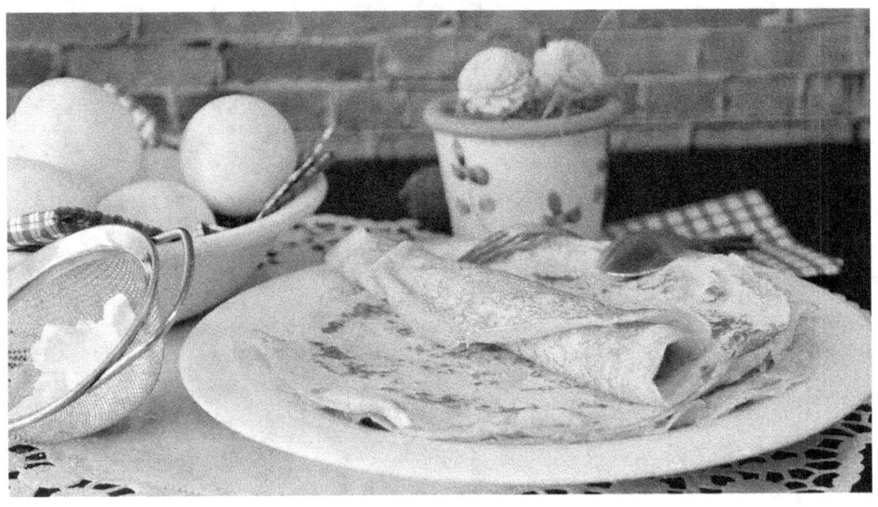

Chapter 4

The Impact of Ultra-processed Foods on Human Health

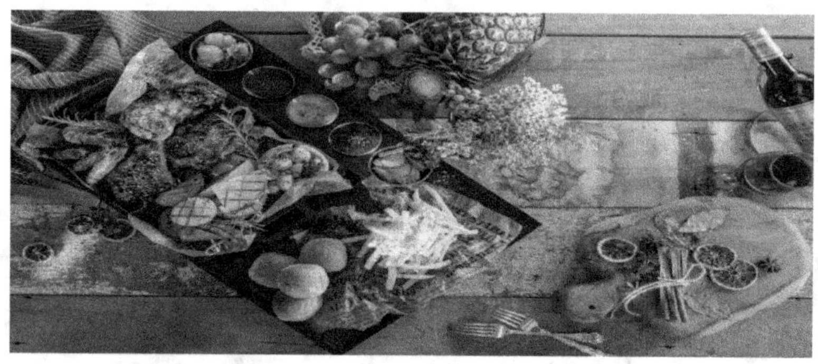

One of the most important public health issues of our day is obesity and metabolic disorders, of which eating a lot of highly processed food is a major contributing cause. The intricate connection between these health issues and ultra-processed diets is examined below:

1) OBESITY:

- **Caloric Density:** Ultra-processed foods are generally poor in vital nutrients and excessive in calories. These foods often include high-calorie content per gram of food, which makes them energy-dense and may lead to overconsumption and weight gain.

- **High Sugar and Fat Content:** Several ultra-processed foods are loaded with added sugars as well as unhealthy fats such as trans and saturated fats. Overconsumption of these ingredients might result in obesity and weight gain due to their tendency to cause an imbalance between energy intake and expenditure.

- ☐ **InsufficUltra-processed** foods are often dietary fiber and protein and these are crucial for fostering sensations of fullness and satisfaction. Consequently, people ultra-processed food in greater amounts without feeling satisfied, which might eventually lead to overeating and weight gain.

- ☐ **Impact on Eating Behaviours:** Ultra-processed foods' hyper palatability, together with their extensive availability and aggressive marketing, might encourage excessive consumption and unhealthy eating habits. These meals are designed to be highly rewarding and addictive, which may cause overindulgence and cravings, especially in more vulnerable individuals.

2) Metabolic Disorders:

- ☐ **Insulin Resistance**: Ultraprocessed feature diets, particularly those heavy in refined sugacarbohydratesydrates, may lead to insulin resistance, which is a guarantee of metabolic disorders like type 2 diabetes. Insulin resistance is a condition in which cells lose their ability to respond to the effects of insulin leading to a rise in blood sugar levels and an increase in insulin produced by the pancreas.

- ☐ **Dyslipidemia:** Ultra-processed foods usually contain high levels of unhealthy fats, such as trans and saturated fats which can be a contributing factor to dyslipidemia, an abnormal lipid profile marked by decreased levels of HDL cholesterol (the "good" cholesterol) and elevated levels of LDL cholesterol (the "bad" cholesterol). Dyslipidemia is one of the main risk factors for metabolic and cardiovascular diseases.

☐ **Inflammation and Oxidative Stress:** Ultra-processed food intake has been connected to elevated levels of oxidative stress and inflammation in the body, which are fundamental processes associated with the development of metabolic diseases as mentioned earlier. Ultra-processed meals containing large amounts of harmful fats, refined sugars, and additives make it to promote inflammation and oxidative damage, leading to metabolic dysfunction.

☐ **Gut Microbiota Dysbiosis:** Emerging research suggests that eating a lot of processed food may have a detrimental effect on the diversity and composition of the gut microbiota, resulting in dysbiosis, or an imbalance in the gut bacteria. Dysbiosis has been linked to metabolic disorders such as obesity, and insulin resistance among others suggesting a possible role for gut health in metabolic health.

3) Cardiovascular Health:

A vital component of total health is cardiovascular health, and eating a diet high in processed foods hurts it. Let's examine the intricate connection between ultra-processed meals and cardiovascular disease.

☐ **High Levels of Unhealthy Fats:**

Saturated and Trans Fats: Trans fats are created via the hydrogenation process, which solidifies liquid vegetable oils and has been discussed earlier to be present in ultra-processed foods. The risk of atherosclerosis and cardiovascular disease is increased by trans fats which are known to raise levels of "bad" cholesterol (LDL) and lower levels of "good" cholesterol (HDL).

☐ Excessive Sodium Intake:

Processed and Packaged Foods: Ultra-processed foods are a significant source of dietary sodium because they often contain added salt for flavor enhancement and preservation. Excessive salt consumption may cause greater fluid retention and put stress on the heart and blood vessels, it is linked to hypertension, or high blood pressure, which is a key risk factor for cardiovascular disease.

☐ Added sugars and refined carbohydrates:

High Index of Glycemia: The refined carbohydrates and added sugars used in many ultra-processed meals have a high glycemic index which has been connected to inflammation, dyslipidemia, and insulin resistance—all of which are cardiovascular disease risk factors.

☐ Low Density of Nutrients:

Many Nutrients: Diets deficient in essential nutrients raise the risk of heart disease and stroke and may worsen cardiovascular health.

☐ Oxidative stress and inflammation:

The main causes of cardiovascular disease include oxidative stress and chronic inflammation, which also lead to endothelial dysfunction, the development of arterial plaque, and atherosclerosis.

☐ Effect on Obesity and Weight

4) The Risk of Cancer

Cancer is a highly complex and multifaceted disease influenced by a wide range of factors such as the individual's lifestyle, environmental, and hereditary variables. Although research on the precise mechanisms relating ultra-processed foods to cancer risk is still ongoing, some factors point to a possible correlation. Let's explore the comprehensive knowledge of how increased consumption of ultra-processed food may increase your risk of cancer.

a) Preservatives and Additives:

- **Sulfur and Nitrites:** Hot dogs, bacon, and deli meats are examples of ultra-processed meats that often use nitrates and nitrites as preservatives. These substances can combine with amino acids during high-temperature cooking methods like grilling or frying to create nitrosamines, which are recognized carcinogens connected to some malignancies, including stomach and colorectal cancers.

- **Artificial Colors and flavors:** Ultra-processed foods contain artificial colors and flavors that have been implicated as potential carcinogens. For instance, research on animals has connected several artificial food colors, such as Red 40 and Yellow 5, to a higher risk of cancer.

b) Unhealthy Fats:

- **Trans Fats:** Trans fats have been linked to a higher chance of developing several malignancies, such as prostate and breast cancer.

c) High Glycemic Index Carbohydrates:

- **IGF (insulin-like growth factor) and insulin:** High quantities of added sugars and refined carbohydrates as discussed earlier may raise insulin and insulin-like growth factor (IGF) levels. Due to their ability to stimulate cell division and growth, these hormones have been linked to the initiation and spread of cancer.

d) Oxidative stress and inflammation:

- **Refined Substances:** Preservatives, chemicals, and processed substances included in many ultra-processed meals may cause oxidative stress and inflammation in the body. It is thought that oxidative stress and chronic inflammation contribute to the development of cancer by causing DNA damage and encouraging the growth of tumors.

e) Disruption of Gut Microbiota:

- Dysbiosis: Recent studies indicate that ultra-processed foods may disrupt the gut microbiota's equilibrium and cause dysbiosis, which is an imbalance in the composition of the gut bacteria. Therefore, increased oxidative stress and inflammation in the gut have been related to dysbiosis and may contribute to the development of cancer.

f) High Caloric Density and Obesity:

- **Obesity-Related Cancers:** Ultra-processed food diets are rich in calories and may lead to weight gain and obesity. Breast, endometrial, and colorectal cancers are among the cancers for which obesity is a recognized risk factor.

5) Effects on Mental Health

It is important to comprehend how ultra-processed foods affect mental health since our dietary choices influence significantly our psychological well-being. Let's explore the whole knowledge of the potential impact of ultra-processed meals on mental health.

a) Nutrient Deficiencies:

- **Micronutrients imbalance:** Ultra-processed foods are deficient in essential nutrients such as vitamins, minerals, and antioxidants which can result in deficits in important nutrients such as magnesium, omega-3 fatty acids, B vitamins, and vitamin D that are critical for health and proper function of the brain.

- **Impact on Neurotransmitters:** Neurotransmitters play a vital role in controlling mood, cognition, and behavior. Nutrient deficiencies resulting from the production and consumption of ultra-processed foods can disrupt the balance of these natural neurotransmitters resulting in difficulties for serotonin, dopamine, and gamma-aminobutyric acid (GABA) to perform their normal functions.. An imbalance in these neurotransmitters has been connected to mental health conditions including depression, anxiety, and attention deficit hyperactivity disorder (ADHD).

b) Inflammation and Oxidative stress:

- **Processed Ingredients:** Ultra Processed meals are generally loaded with additives, preservatives, and processed ingredients that may promote oxidative stress and inflammation in the body. However, chronic inflammation and oxidative stress have been reported to be contributing factors to several mental health conditions, such as anxiety, depression, and neurodegenerative diseases like Alzheimer's and Parkinson's disease.

c) Gut-brain Axis Dysfunction:

☐ **Effect on the Gut Microbiota:** Dysbiosis about ultraprocessed foods as discussed earlier has been linked to alterations in brain function and behavior through the gut-brain axis, a two-way communication channel between the gut and the brain. Imbalances in the gut microbiota have been linked to a higher risk of mental health disorders such as anxiety, depression, and autism spectrum disorders.

d) Sugar and Mood Swings:

☐ **Dysregulation of Blood Sugar:** Ultra-processed meals heavy in refined sugars may cause rapid fluctuations in blood sugar levels, which can cause fatigue, irritability, and mood swings. These fluctuations have the potential to disrupt neurotransmitter function and worsen the symptoms of mental illnesses like anxiety and depression.

e) Behavioral Effects:

☐ **Addictive Characteristics**: Ultra-processed foods are often designed to be very appealing and addictive, activating the reward regions in the brain thereby encouraging cravings and compulsive eating habits. Overindulgence in these foods may result in emotional eating, dysregulated eating behaviors, and food addiction—all of which are associated with poor mental health outcomes.

f) Cognitive Impairment:

☐ **Brain Fog:** Ultraprocessed food diets have been linked to cognitive impairment, which includes poor memory, concentration difficulties, and impaired cognitive function. Ultra-processed foods have oxidative and inflammatory properties that, when combined with nutrient deficits, may damage the brain and cause cognitive decline over time.

Chapter 5

Socioeconomic and Environmental Consequences

A) Economic Costs and Burdens

Ultra-processed foods have a variety of economic costs and burdens on individuals, communities, and societies. These expenses go beyond the price tag of the groceries and may have a significant consequence on productivity, environmental sustainability, public health, and healthcare systems.

1) Healthcare Costs:

- ☐ **Chronic Diseases:** Ultra-processed foods are a major cause of some chronic and terminal diseases due to their composition. Therefore, healthcare systems have a heavy burden in managing and treating chronic illnesses.

- ☐ **Healthcare Expenditure:** Medical consultations, hospital stays, prescription drugs, and surgery are among the major healthcare expenses associated with treating diet-related disorders. These costs put pressure on both public and private healthcare budgets and may result in increased individual insurance rates.

2) Productivity Loss:

- **Absenteeism and Presenteeism:** Poor dietary habits associated with consuming highly processed foods might result in a rise in absenteeism (sick leave) and a reduction in productivity when working (presenteeism). Workers' performance and efficiency may be impacted by fatigue, lack of concentration, and diminished cognitive function.

- **Workplace Wellness Programs:** Employers may have to incur expenses for the implementation of wellness initiatives such as education campaigns, subsidized healthy food options, and fitness programs, to encourage healthy eating habits among the employees.

3) Environmental Costs:

- **Depletion of Resources:** The manufacture of ultra-processed foods normally depends on intense agricultural methods which degrades soil, pollutes water, destroys forests, and reduces biodiversity. This strains natural resources and ecosystems, requiring expensive environmental conservation and remediation measures.

- **Climate Change:** Industrial food processing and transportation both increase greenhouse gas emissions, which exacerbate climate change. It will entail high economic costs to invest in renewable energy, sustainable agriculture, and carbon offsetting strategies to mitigate these emissions.

4) Subsidies and Externalities:

- **Government Subsidies:** The cultivation of commodities like maize and soybeans that are used in ultra-processed meals may be encouraged by agricultural subsidies, which might skew market pricing and keep unhealthy food options affordable.

☐ **Externalities:** The negative externalities such as healthcare costs and environmental damages that are associated with ultra-processed foods are not often reflected in their market prices. This later leads to inefficiencies or even market failure since society bears the true costs instead of producers and consumers.

5) Social Welfare and Inequality:

☐ **Food Insecurity:** Ultra-processed foods are cheaper and readily available than fresh, whole-nutrient alternatives, contributing to malnourishment and food insecurity, especially among low-income populations. This places additional burdens on Charity organizations and social welfare institutions.

☐ **Health Disparities:** Consumption patterns of ultra-processed foods contribute to health disparities in a case whereby disadvantaged populations have limited access to inexpensive, healthy food alternatives which disproportionately impact them with diet-related illnesses. Public health initiatives and targeted interventions are needed to address these discrepancies.

6) Regulatory and Policy Costs:

☐ **Food Regulation:** Governments incur costs to create and implement laws about nutritional standards, food safety, labeling, and advertising. To encourage better eating choices, policymakers may impose taxes, subsidies, or limits on ultra-processed foods. However, doing so may result in administrative expenses and regulatory compliance challenges for companies.

☐ **Public Health Campaigns:** Public education campaigns are designed to increase public awareness of the health concerns connected with ultra-processed foods. This will require adequate funding and resources to develop and disseminate the informational materials via a variety of channels.

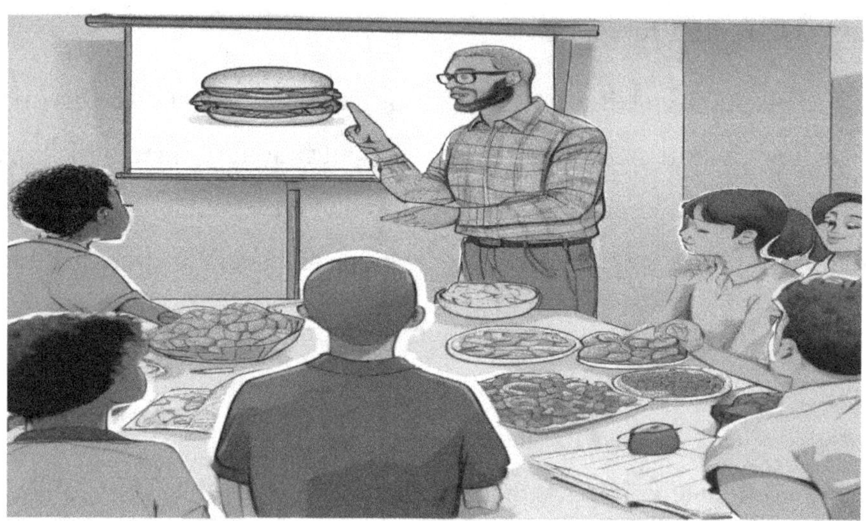

B) Environmental Footprint of Ultra-processed Foods

Comprehending the ecological impact of highly processed meals is crucial to tackling sustainability issues related to food production and consumption. Now let's explore the whole knowledge of the impacts of ultra-processed foods on the environment.

1) Production Requires a Lot of Resources:

- **Use of Land:** Large amounts of land are often required for the agricultural production of raw materials such as crops like maize, soybeans, and wheat, as well as cattle for the production of meat and dairy products for ultra-processed meals. Expansion of agricultural land used for the production of ultra-processed food may result in deforestation, habitat destruction, biodiversity loss, and soil degradation.

- **Use of Water:** The massive production of Ultra-processed foods requires significant volumes of water for irrigation, processing, and cleaning. Furthermore, Water-intensive crops such as a result of maize and soybeans that are commonly utilized in ultra-processed meals, may exacerbate the problem of water scarcity, especially in regions that are experiencing drought conditions or have restricted water supply.

2) Energy Consumption and Greenhouse Gas Emissions:

☐ **Processing and Manufacturing:** The processing and manufacturing of ultra-processed food items require a substantial amount of energy consumption for machinery operation, heating, cooling, and transportation. Fossil fuel reliance is a contributing factor to greenhouse gas emissions, which are the main causes of climate change. These emissions include carbon dioxide (CO_2), methane (CH_4), and nitrous oxide (N_2O).

☐ **Transportation and Packaging:** Ultra-processed meals are often packed in single-use plastic wrappers, containers, and packaging materials, which adds to plastic pollution and deteriorates the environment. Furthermore, the long-distance transportation of highly processed goods from manufacturing sites to distribution centers and retail outlets increases energy consumption and greenhouse gas emissions.

3) Food Waste and Losses:

☐ **Supply Chain Waste:** Ultra-processed foods have a high potential for food waste and losses throughout the supply chain, including during harvesting, processing, packing, shipping, and retail. Food waste is a contributing factor to greenhouse gas emissions, contamination of the environment, and wasteful use of labor, water, energy, and land.

4) Effect on Ecosystems and Biodiversity:

☐ **Monoculture Farming:** Monoculture farming methods, which include the cultivation of a single crop across enormous expanses of land, are often used in the intense production of raw materials for ultra-processed meals. Monoculture farming may cause ecosystems to be disrupted and decrease biodiversity via erosion, fertilizer runoff, soil depletion, and loss of natural plants.

☐ **Use of Herbicides and Pesticides:** Synthetic pesticides and herbicides are used extensively in the manufacturing of ultra-processed food to control pests, weeds, and diseases. The extensive use of agrochemicals may affect non-target organisms including pollinators, birds, and aquatic species, as well as have detrimental effects on biodiversity, soil health, and water quality.

5) Fairness in Social and Environmental Spheres:

☐ **Environmental Inequalities:** The environmental effects of ultra-processed foods are frequently unequally distributed, with low-income groups, people of color, and marginalized communities suffering disproportionately from water contamination, land degradation, pollution, and climate change-related disasters linked to food processing and production facilities.

C) Social Justice and Inequality in the Context of Ultra-Processed Foods

Social justice and inequality are closely linked to the manufacturing, distribution, and consumption of ultra-processed foods, with vulnerable people bearing a disproportionate share of the negative impacts of these foods. Let's explore the whole knowledge of how highly processed meals fuel inequality and social injustice:

1) Availability and Accessibility:

- **Food Deserts:** Low-income areas and communities of color, where access to fresh, healthy meals is limited (often known as "food deserts") are majorly the places where ultra-processed foods are more easily found and affordable. The scarcity of grocery shops, farmers' markets, and other healthy food alternatives in these areas force locals to depend on ultra-processed meals sold mostly at convenience stores, fast food joints, and corner stores.

- **Access to Healthy Food:** Limited availability of wholesome, minimally processed foods in Food deserts results in disparities in diet quality and nutrition-related health consequences, such as increased prevalence of obesity, diabetes, and cardiovascular disease among people. In marginalized communities, the lack of access to nutritious food feeds the cycles of poverty and poor health, aggravating social injustices.

2) Marketing and Targeting Groups:

- **Predatory Marketing:** Ultra-processed food industries often target vulnerable groups, such as children, adolescents, and communities of color through aggressive marketing strategies. These marketing techniques promote unhealthy foods relative referred to as ultraprocessed foods leading to overindulgence and bad eating habits among these selected populations.

- **Cultural Appropriation:** Ultra-processed food industries regularly appropriate ethnic symbols, traditions, and identities to market their products to certain demographic groups, thereby reinforcing stereotypes and perpetuating cultural appropriation. This exploitation of cultural heritage further marginalized communities and reinforces inequality in the food system.

3) Labor Exploitation:

- **Low-Wage Workers:** The production and processing of ultra-processed foods depend heavily on a vast network of low-wage workers, including farm laborers, factory workers, and food service employees, many of whom are immigrants, people of color, and women. These workers often endure exploitative working circumstances that contribute to social injustice and economic inequality. These conditions include long hours, low wages, a lack of benefits, and exposure to hazardous chemicals.

Chapter 6

Consumer Behavior and Food Choices

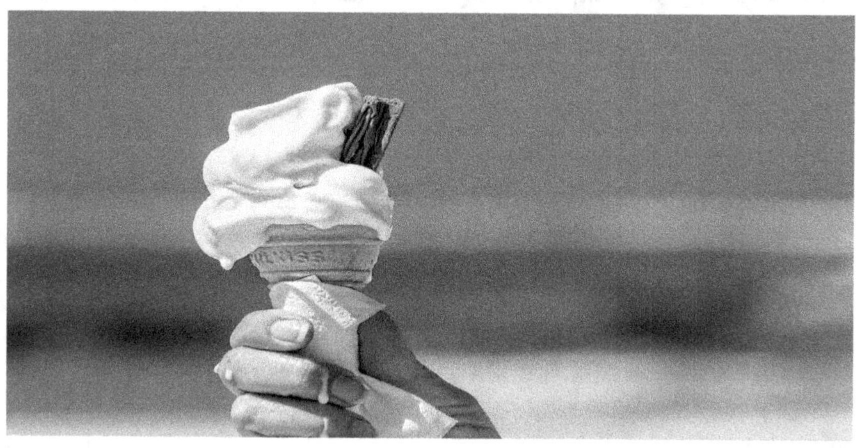

Psychological Factors Influencing Consumption Ultra-processed Foods

The consumption of ultra-processed meals is influenced by numerous psychological elements that impact people's eating habits and food choices. It is essential to understand these psychological factors to create treatments that effectively encourage better eating habits. Now let's investigate in detail the psychological aspects that impact the eating of highly processed foods:

1) Palatability and Cravings:

- **Food Reward System:** Ultraprocessed meals are often designed to be very rewarding and palatable, activating the brain's reward system and triggering feelings of satisfaction and pleasure. These meals are hard to resist and encourage cravings and overindulgence since they are designed to appeal to our natural inclinations for sweet, salty, and fatty tastes.

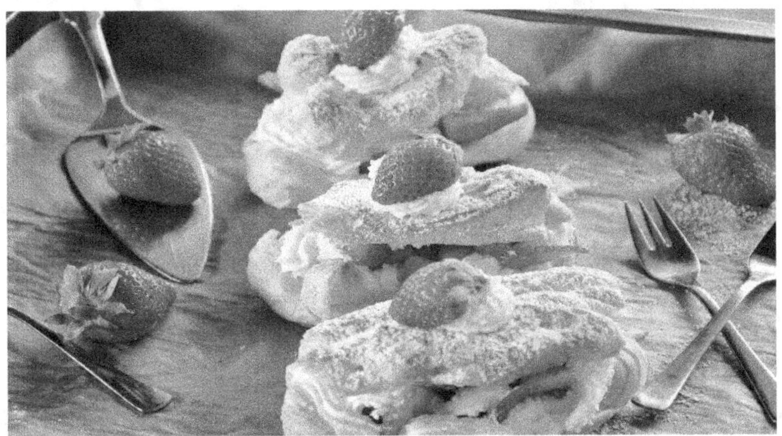

- **Conditioned Responses:** Repetitive exposure to ultra-processed foods may cause conditioned responses and cravings, as the brain links meals to feelings of reward and pleasure. Environmental signals such as food advertisements, packaging, and availability might promote these urges and encourage ultra-processed food intake as a habit.

2) Emotional Consumption:

- **Stress and Negative Feelings:** Ultraprocessed meals are a common coping mechanism used by individuals to cope with stress, negative emotions, boredom, or loneliness. Emotional eating offers momentary relief from unpleasant emotions and has the potential to develop into a habitual response to emotional stimuli, resulting in an excessive intake of comfort foods that are high in calories.

- **Reward and Comfort:** Ultra-processed foods provide a momentary escape from mental suffering and are often associated with sentiments of pleasure, feelings of comfort, and nostalgia. Emotional eating habits may be strengthened by the sensory qualities such as taste, texture, and scent of these foods, which can arouse positive feelings and create a sense of pleasure and satisfaction.

3) Convenience and Accessibility:

☐ **Time Constraints:** People with hectic schedules and little free time may choose ready-to-eat ultra-processed meals that are easy to prepare and require little effort. Convenience meals provide individuals with a quick and easy solution for mealtime problems, saving them time and energy without compromising flavor or satisfaction.

☐ **Availability and Marketing:**

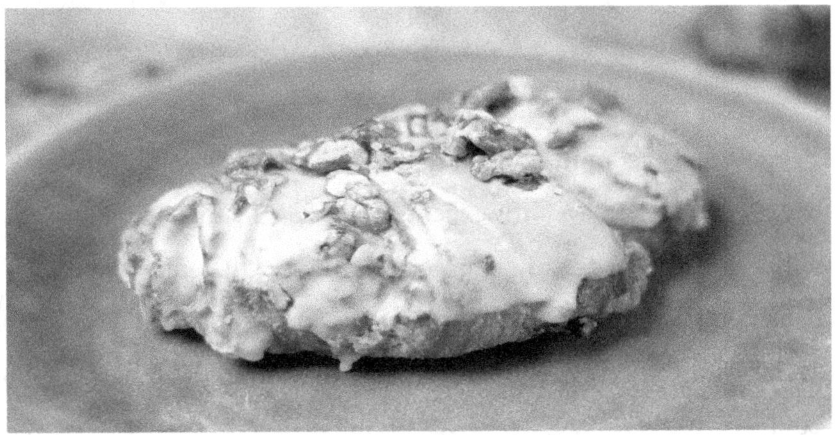

Ultra-processed foods are easily found in our environment, and readily available at supermarkets, convenience stores, fast-food restaurants, and vending machines. The widespread marketing and advertising of these foods promote their accessibility and appeal, which makes them a desirable option for those looking for quick satisfaction and convenience.

4) Social Influences:

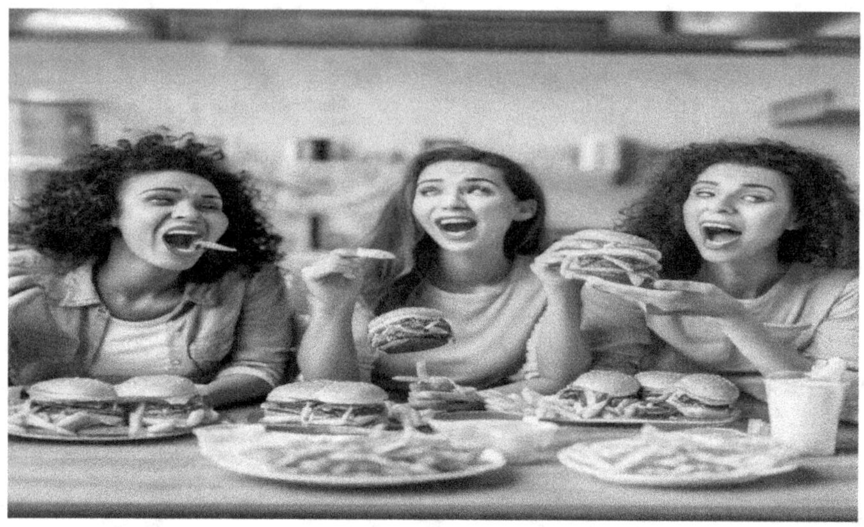

- **Peer pressure and Social Norms:** People's eating habits and food preferences may be influenced by social factors such as peer pressure, cultural influences, and social conventions. Ultra-processed foods are often consumed during social gatherings, celebrations, and communal meals, thereby reinforcing their acceptance and normalization within social contexts.

- **Family and Childhood Experiences:** Family dynamics, parental feeding methods, and childhood food experiences may have a long-term influence on an individual's dietary choices and eating habits. Growing up in environments where ultra-processed foods are regularly consumed and rewarded can influence taste preferences, portion sizes, and food attitudes into adulthood.

5) Cognitive Biases:

☐ **Food Perceptions and Beliefs:** Individual's perceptions and beliefs about food might influence their food choices and behaviors. Also, ultra-processed meals might be overeaten due to cognitive biases like the "health halo effect" (perceiving unhealthy foods as healthy based on specific qualities) or the "licensing effect" (compensating for good food choices by indulging in harmful ones).

☐ **Temporal Discounting:** Despite the possible long-term detrimental impacts on health and well-being, individuals may still opt for ultra-processed meals to provide instant pleasure and satisfaction above the long-term health concerns.

Marketing Techniques Used in the Ultra-processed Food Sector

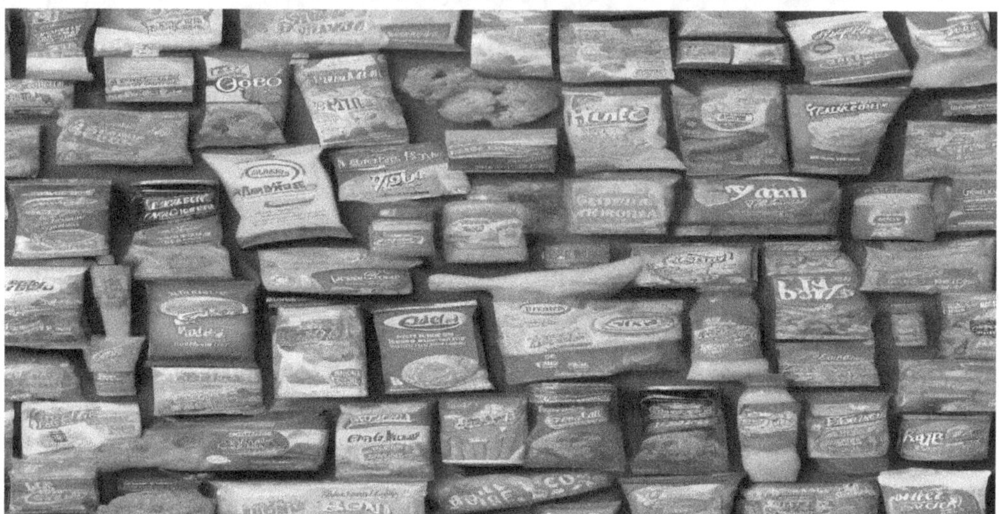

The ultra-processed food industry uses a range of advanced marketing techniques to advertise its products, target certain consumer demographics, and increase sales and profits. These techniques use consumer behavior research, psychological concepts, and advanced advertising methods to influence consumers' opinions and judgments about what to buy. Now let us take a closer look at the marketing techniques used by the ultra-processed food industry:

1) Targeted Advertising:

- **Demographic Targeting:** Ultra-processed food companies select target audiences based on factors like age, gender, income level, and lifestyle choices by using consumer segmentation strategies and demographic data. Companies may successfully reach and engage their target customers by customizing their product offers and advertising appeal messages to certain demographic groups.

☐ **Digital Marketing:** The emergence of internet platforms and digital media has completely changed the marketing of ultra-processed food. Companies use influencer marketing, social media, SEO, and targeted online advertising to connect with consumers via a variety of digital platforms and channels.

2) Branding and Product Positioning:

☐ **Brand Recognition:** Companies that produce ultra-processed foods make significant investments in creating powerful brands that are well-known and have favorable connotations. Companies meticulously compose their slogans, mascots, package designs, and logos to build brand identification and customer loyalty.

☐ **Health and Wellness Claims:** Health and wellness claims, such as "low-fat," "sugar-free," "natural," or "organic," are often used in the marketing of ultra-processed food items in an attempt to appeal to health-conscious consumers. Even though these statements could be misleading or exaggerated, they create the perception of healthier alternatives and increase sales.

3) Product Innovation and Variety:

☐ **Development of New Products:** Ultra-processed food companies that produce ultra-processed food constantly develop and launch new goods to adapt to changing consumer demands and industry trends. Product development teams use customer surveys, market research, and taste testing to find new trends and produce food items that are appealing to consumers.

□ **Flavor and Texture Optimization:** Ultra-Processed Foods are meticulously designed to satisfy customers' senses of taste, texture, fragrance, and mouthfeel. Also, food scientists use flavor enhancers, texturizers, and other additives to improve a product's sensory qualities and enhance their palatability.

4) Promotional Techniques:

□ **Price Promotions:** Ultra-processed food manufacturers employ price promotions, discounts, coupons, and exclusive deals to entice customers to buy their goods. Price promotions create a sense of urgency among consumers and promote impulsive purchases.

□ **Cross-Promotions:** Ultra-processed food manufacturers often work with other brands, retailers, or media organizations to expand and promote their product lines and reach new audiences. Product placements sponsored content, and co-branded promotions all aid in raising brand awareness and boosting sales.

5) Emotional Appealing and Storytelling:

□ **Emotional Branding:** Manufacturers of ultra-processed foods use emotional appeals and storytelling techniques to make an emotional connection with customers and arouse good memories or sentiments connected to their products. To emotionally connect customers, advertisements often involve familiar personalities, endearing tales, or nostalgic themes.

- ☐ **Aspirational Lifestyle:** Ultra-processed food advertisements often feature idealized lifestyles, aspirations, and social interactions connected to the consumption of their products. Images of happy families, social gatherings, and outdoor adventures convey feelings of contentment, pleasure, and fulfillment that consumers want to achieve via their purchases.

6) Influencer Marketing:

- ☐ **Social Media Influencers:** Ultra-processed food firms work with bloggers, celebrities, and content producers on social media to market their products to a larger audience. Influencers approve items and use their reputation and power to change the perceptions and actions of their consumers through sponsored posts, product reviews, and brand collaborations.

Strategies for Behavioral Change for Ultra-Processed Foods

It takes a multidimensional strategy that takes into account systemic issues, environmental effects, cultural norms, and individual preferences to change behaviors linked to the intake of ultra-processed foods. Now let's go deep into the analysis of several approaches to changing behavior about ultra-processed foods:

1) Knowledge and Consciousness:

- **Nutrition Education:** Giving people accurate and easily available information on the health impacts, nutritional makeup, and processing techniques of ultra-processed foods may enable them to make well-informed dietary decisions. Programs, seminars, and materials dedicated to nutrition education may help spread the word about the possible dangers of consuming too many ultra-processed foods and encourage the use of healthier alternatives.

- **Labeling and Transparency:** Consumers may identify ultra-processed foods and make better decisions by using clear and informative food labeling, such as ingredient lists, nutrition information panels, and front-of-package labels. Encouraging openness in food labeling and advertising may boost customer confidence and help with well-informed decision-making.

2) Encouraging Whole, Minimally Processed, Foods:

- **Encouraging Cooking Skills:** People may take charge of their diets and lessen their dependency on highly processed foods by learning how to prepare simple, affordable, and nutritious meals using whole, minimally processed foods. Building cooking abilities and confidence in the kitchen

☐ may be facilitated by cooking workshops, recipe demonstrations, and online tutorials.

☐ **Increasing Access to Healthy Foods:** Making it simpler for people to include nutrient-dense options in their diets and lessen their dependency on highly processed foods can be accomplished by expanding access to fresh, whole foods through programs like farmers' markets, community gardens, urban agriculture projects, and mobile food markets.

3) Behavioral Nudges and Environmental Changes:

☐ **Healthy Defaults:** Changing the environment around food to support healthy defaults, such as serving water in place of sugary drinks or arranging fruits and vegetables at eye level in grocery stores, may promote better eating choices without limiting personal freedom.

☐ **Portion Control:** Reducing overconsumption and encouraging mindful eating behaviors may be achieved by putting portion control measures into practice, such as providing reduced portion sizes or packing ultra-processed foods in single-serving containers.

4) Social and Community Support:

Peer Support Groups: Establishing encouraging settings where people may interact with others who have similar dietary and health objectives can provide accountability, inspiration, and motivation. Online forums, community-based initiatives, and peer support groups may all help with behavior modification techniques, recipe exchanges, and information sharing.

Cultural and Social Norms: Changing societal attitudes and behaviors around food consumption may be achieved by promoting cultural traditions, values, and social norms that place a higher priority on whole, minimally processed foods. Encouraging culinary customs that are based on sustainability and health as well as celebrating ethnic variety, may strengthen social bonds and promote wholesome eating habits.

5) Environmental and Policy Interventions:

- **Food Policy Advocacy:** Fighting for laws that promote healthy eating environments, such as those requiring nutrition labels, prohibiting the marketing of unhealthy foods to minors, and providing subsidies for fruits and vegetables, can lead to structural adjustments that encourage eating a more balanced diet and lower consumption of highly processed foods.

- **Regulatory Measures:** Putting rules and regulations into place to restrict the marketing, availability, and accessibility of ultra-processed meals in public spaces such as workplaces, schools, and parks may contribute to the development of environments that support health and well-being. Limiting the availability of highly processed meals in cafeterias, vending machines, and recreational establishments may help reduce exposure and temptation.

Chapter 7

Regulatory Framework and Policy Responses

Current Regulations and Supervision for Ultra-processed Foods

To promote food safety, transparency, and public health, a complex interaction between industry standards, government laws, and consumer advocacy initiatives is involved in the regulation of ultra-processed foods. Let's take a close look at the legislative structure and policy measures controlling ultra-processed foods:

1) Food Labeling and Nutritional Standards:

- **Nutrition Labeling Requirements:** Many countries have imposed regulations that make the manufacturers provide comprehensive nutritional information on food labels, including serving sizes, calorie contents, and levels of essential elements like fat, sugar, salt, and additives. Well-clear and detailed informative labeling assist consumers in making informed decisions and understanding the nutritional content of ultra-processed foods.

- **Front-of-Package Labeling:** Some countries have put in place front-of-package labeling systems to highlight the nutritional quality of foods and beverages. These labels use color-coded symbols, logos, or numerical ratings to show if a food satisfies certain nutritional standards or exceeds recommended ingredients like sugar, salt, or saturated fat.

2) Restrictions of Advertising and Marketing:

- ☐ **Marketing to Children:** Several nations have laws that prohibit the marketing of ultra-processed foods to children, especially via the Internet, television, and other media. These rules are meant to shield children from the effects of deceptive advertising and encourage healthier food choices.

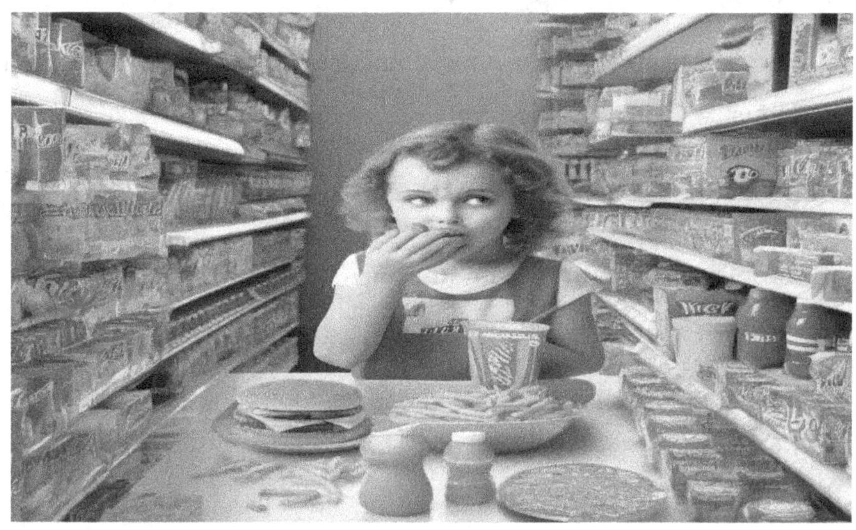

- ☐ **Health Claims and Misleading Advertising:** Regulatory bodies often impose rules for health claims and advertising practices to stop deceptive or misleading marketing strategies. It may be necessary for companies to provide substantial evidence to support their claims on the nutritional value or health advantages of their products and to avoid making false or inflated claims.

3) Food Safety Regulations:

- **Food Additives and Preservatives:** A range of additives, preservatives, and flavor enhancers are often added to ultra-processed foods as described earlier. Regulatory Agencies have set maximum limits and safety standards for the ingestion of these additives to guarantee that they are safe for consumption and do not pose health risks to consumers.

- **Contaminant Limits:** To safeguard the public's health, regulations establish limits for dangerous pollutants such as heavy metals, pesticides, and microbiological infections in food items. Frequent testing, inspection, and monitoring programs help in identifying possible consumer hazards and ensuring adherence to safety regulations.

4) Dietary Guidelines and Public Health Campaigns:

- **National Dietary Guidelines:** To encourage wholesome eating and avoid illnesses linked to nutrition, governments provide dietary guidelines and recommendations. These recommendations emphasize whole, minimally processed meals and discourage the use of ultra-processed foods that are rich in harmful fats, sugars, and chemicals. They provide evidence-based guidance on food choices, portion sizes, and nutrient intake.

- **Public Health Campaigns:** Public health authorities and non-profit organizations run educational campaigns and initiatives to encourage healthy eating habits and increase knowledge of the health concerns associated with excessive consumption of ultra-processed foods. To reach a large variety of audiences and promote behavior change, these campaigns may make use of online resources, school programs, community events, and media outreach.

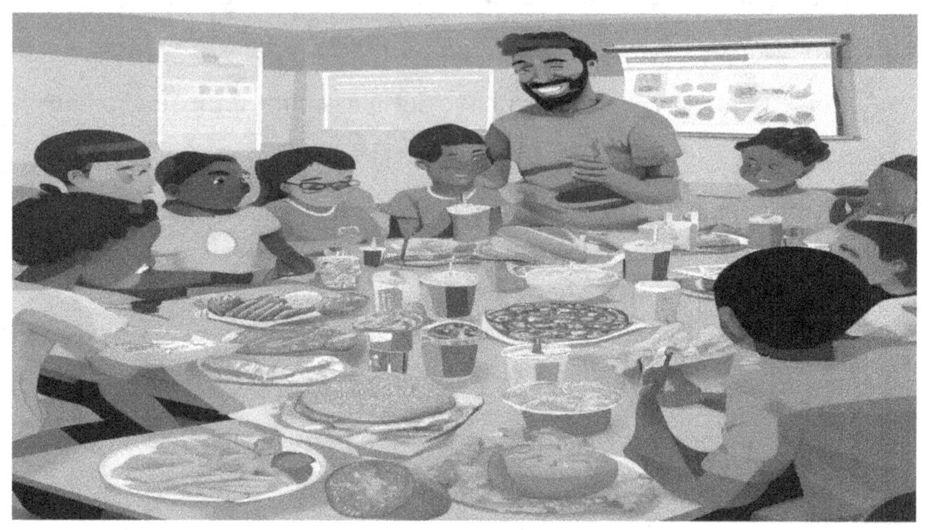

5) International Trade Agreements and Standards:

☐ **Codex Alimentarius:** The Food and Agriculture Organization (FAO) and the World Health Organization (WHO) of the United Nations established the Codex Alimentarius Commission to provide global guidelines for food safety, quality, and labeling. These standards provide a foundation for standardizing laws and promoting global commerce in food items, especially highly processed foods.

☐ **Trade Agreements:** Trade Agreements between nations may have an influence on laws controlling ultra-processed goods, especially those about market access, food safety rules, and labeling specifications. The goal of negotiations and agreements is to strike a balance between public health goals and trade interests, as well as to make sure that regulatory actions comply with international commitments and standards.

6) Lobbying and Advocacy Activities

1) Studies and Policy Evaluation:

- ☐ **Evidence-Based Advocacy:** To provide information on the health effects of ultra-processed foods and to influence policy talks and decision-making procedures, advocacy organizations carry out research and policy analysis. Advocacy organizations may impact the creation of evidence-based laws and regulations that prioritize public health by supplying legislators with reliable data and analysis.

- ☐ **Monitoring and Evaluation:** Advocacy organizations keep an eye on how ultra-processed food rules are implemented and enforced, as well as how well they address public health issues. This continuous assessment and monitoring aid in discovering weak points in the way policies are being implemented, difficulties with enforcement, and areas for development.

2) International Cooperation and Advocacy:

- ☐ **Worldwide Advocacy Efforts:** To address issues including food insecurity, malnutrition, and non-communicable illnesses that are linked to ultra-processed foods, advocacy organizations undertake worldwide advocacy campaigns. Advocacy groups may promote coordinated action and shared solutions to complicated food system concerns by working with governments, international organizations, and civil society groups.

- ☐ **Policy Harmonization:** To guarantee uniformity and coherence in initiatives to address the health effects of ultra-processed foods, advocacy organizations push for harmonized laws and regulations among nations. This might include promoting global consumer protection and public health goals via international agreements, standards, and recommendations.

Possible Measures to Adopt Policy

The issues surrounding ultra-processed foods may be addressed and better eating habits can be encouraged by some possible legislative initiatives. Aspects of the food environment that are targeted by these interventions include labeling, manufacturing, marketing, and consumer education. Let's examine some possible legislative measures about highly processed foods:

1) Front-of-Package Labeling (FOPL):

☐ Standardized front-of-package labeling systems that provide readily comprehensible information on the nutritional value and overall health of food items are to be implemented.

☐ The use of color-coded labels or symbols should be encouraged to show the concentrations of important nutrients, such as sugar, salt, and saturated fat so that customers can quickly make better decisions.

2) Limiting Marketing to Children:

☐ Implementing laws that prohibit the promotion of highly processed foods that are rich in sugar, salt, and harmful fats to children via the internet, television, and other media platforms.

☐ Enforcing limitations on the use of celebrities, cartoon characters, and other persuasive techniques in kid-targeted food advertisements.

3) Pricing and Taxation Policies:

- ☐ Imposing levies or taxes on ultra-processed foods to deter consumption and raise funds for public health programs.

- ☐ Providing subsidies for the production and consumption of nutritious foods, such as fruits, vegetables, and whole grains, to lower their cost and increase consumer accessibility.

4) Regulation of Food Additives and Preservatives:

- ☐ Tightening control and regulation of food additives, flavor enhancers, and preservatives used in ultra-processed foods to guarantee customer safety and no health concerns.

- ☐ Stricter regulations on the use of artificial flavors, colors, and other substances that might be harmful to health, particularly in young children.

4) School Food Policies:

- ☐ Putting into practice rules and regulations for school lunches that restrict access to highly processed foods heavy in sugar, salt, and harmful fats and emphasize whole, minimally processed foods.

- ☐ Encouraging nutrition instruction and cooking classes in schools to enable pupils to choose better foods and form a lifetime of healthy eating practices.

5) Urban Planning and Food Environment Policies:

- ☐ Creating settings that encourage healthy food choices by including food availability, cost, and quality in urban planning and development policies.

- ☐ Promoting the creation of community gardens, farmers' markets, and other projects that lessen dependency on highly processed foods and provide access to fresh, locally produced food.

6) Industry Regulation and Corporate Responsibility:

- ☐ Enforcing laws requiring food producers to provide details on the materials, processing techniques, and nutritional value of their goods.

- ☐ Holding food businesses responsible for misleading advertising, making false health claims, and engaging in unethical business actions in connection with the creation and promotion of ultra-processed foods.

7) Initiatives for Education and Public Health:

- ☐ Start public health campaigns and educational programs to encourage better eating habits and increase knowledge of the health concerns associated with consuming excessive amounts of ultra-processed foods.

- ☐ Giving customers access to evidence-based data, tools, and resources so they may choose foods wisely and more skillfully manage the food environment.

Policymakers may establish a favorable regulatory environment that encourages healthier food choices, lowers the use of highly processed foods, and improves public health outcomes by combining various policy initiatives. These interventions have to be thorough, grounded on research, and customized to the unique requirements and environments of various communities and groups.

Chapter 8

Alternatives and Solutions for Ultra-processed Foods

Promoting Whole Foods and Traditional Diets

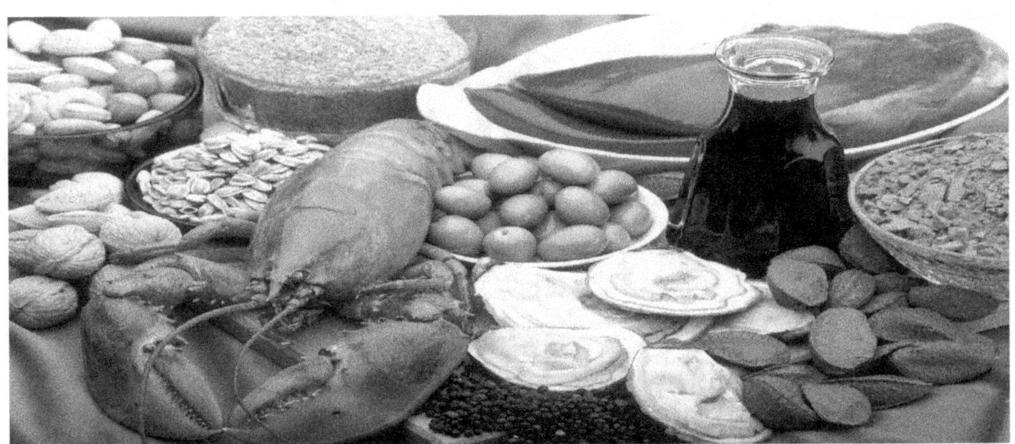

Encouraging whole foods and traditional diets has several advantages that go beyond improving one's health. People may enhance their health, support local food systems, and develop a stronger connection with food and culture by giving priority to minimally processed, nutrient-rich foods that are a part of traditional dietary patterns. Now, let's examine in detail the advantages of endorsing whole foods and conventional diets in place of ultra-processed meals:

1) Health Benefits and Nutritional Quality:

☐ **Density of Nutrients:** Natural sources of vital nutrients such as vitamins, minerals, fiber, and antioxidants include fruits, vegetables, whole grains, legumes, nuts, seeds, and lean meats. Eating a diet high in whole foods gives the body the nutrition it needs to promote immune system function, energy generation, and illness prevention, among other aspects of general health and well-being.

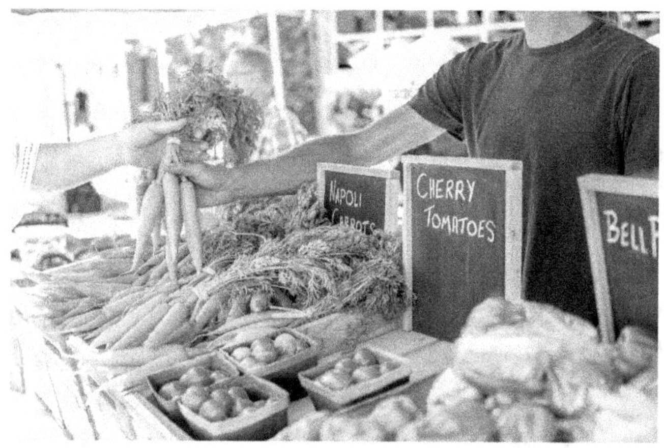

☐ **Prevention of Diseases:** Eating whole foods lowers the chance of developing chronic illnesses including diabetes, obesity, heart disease, and certain types of cancer, among other health advantages. Whole plant meals include phytonutrients, antioxidants, and fiber, which have been shown to have protective benefits against oxidative stress, inflammation, and metabolic abnormalities that are linked to the development of chronic illnesses.

2) Culinary Heritage and Cultural Identity:

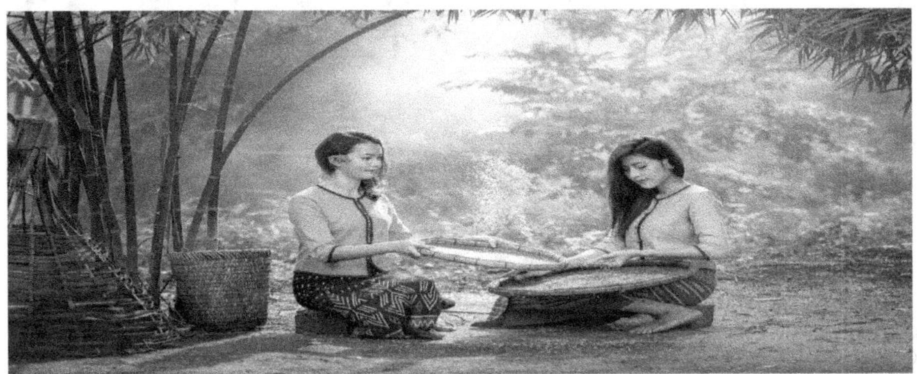

☐ **Preservation of Culinary Traditions:** Customary eating patterns have their roots in gastronomic customs and cultural heritage that have been handed down through the ages. People may establish communal relationships, rediscover their cultural identity, and cultivate a feeling of pride and belonging in their history by conserving and enjoying these culinary traditions.

☐ **Cultural Diversity and Appreciation:** Discovering customary diets from other global cultures introduces individuals to a wide range of tastes, ingredients, and cooking methods. Embracing the diversity of cultures in cuisine encourages respect for various cooking customs as well as unity and understanding across cultural divides.

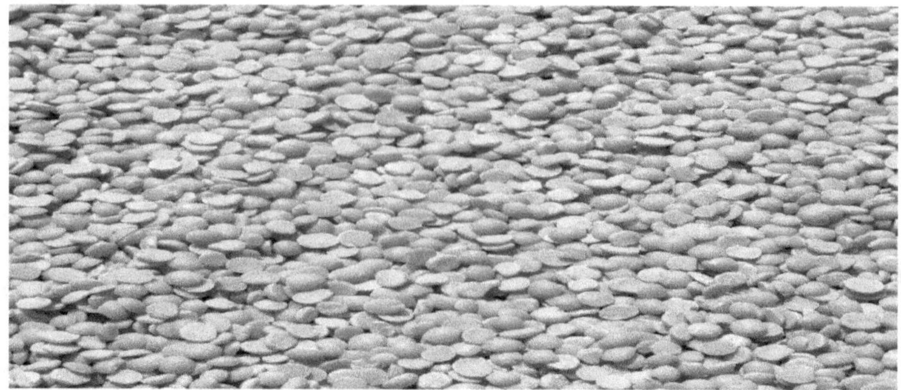

3) Environmental Sustainability:

- **Support for Local Food Systems:** Whole foods are often purchased from nearby farmers and producers to promote sustainable agricultural methods and lessen the environmental impact of food production and delivery. People may lessen their dependency on ultra-processed, mass-produced, and severely processed goods and support the resilience and vitality of their local food systems by buying seasonal, locally farmed food.

- **Reduction of Food Waste:** Traditional diets place a strong emphasis on using whole foods and reduce food waste by preparing meals using every component of the plant or animal. Individuals may lessen food waste and encourage sustainability in their eating habits by using techniques like fermentation, root-to-stem eating, and nose-to-tail cooking.

4) Culinary Enjoyment and Contentment in Food:

- **Flavor and Texture:** The variety of tastes, textures, and scents found in whole foods makes consuming them more pleasurable and fulfilling. Whole foods, from the earthy richness of whole grains to the sweetness of ripe fruits, provide a sensory delight that heavily processed, artificial-flavored products cannot match.

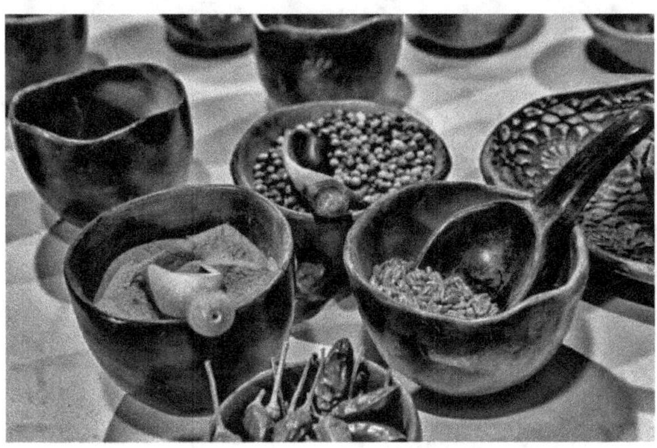

☐ **Cooking Creativity:** Cooking with whole foods promotes exploration and creativity in the kitchen by enabling individuals to explore new novel recipes, ingredients, and cooking techniques. Cooking with whole foods provides endless opportunities for creative and expressive cooking, whether it's fermenting vegetables, baking homemade bread, or making a hearty stew with seasonal veggies.

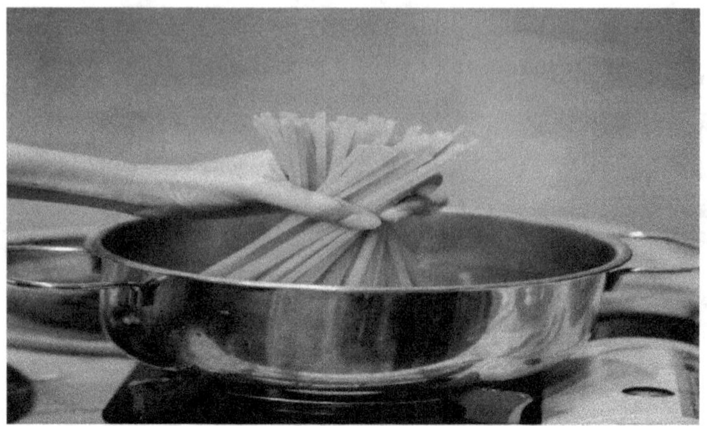

5) Community Well-Being and Social Connection:

- ☐ **Shared Meals and Gatherings:** The value of shared meals and social gatherings as occasions for bonding, celebration, and cross-cultural learning is often emphasized in traditional diets. Eating meals with loved ones, neighbors, and members of the community creates a feeling of community and fortifies social ties, which enhances mental and general well-being.

- ☐ **Support for Local Economies:** Supporting local farmers, artisans, and food producers helps small-scale food businesses flourish while also enhancing the economic health of the communities they live in. Investing in regional food systems promotes a feeling of responsibility and pride in local food traditions and resources while strengthening community resilience.

Food Education and Literacy Initiatives as Remedies for Ultra-processed foods

Food education and literacy initiatives provide a holistic strategy to counteract the ubiquity of highly processed meals by equipping people with the information, abilities, and means to choose better foods. Now let's examine in detail food education and literacy initiatives and their advantages against ultraprocessed foods.

1) Education on Nutrition:

- **Knowing Nutritional Requirements:** Food education initiatives educate people on fundamental nutrition topics, such as the significance of eating a balanced diet full of entire foods including fruits, vegetables, whole grains, lean meats, and healthy fats. To assist them in making decisions and achieving their nutritional goals, participants get information on essential nutrients, portion sizes, and dietary standards.

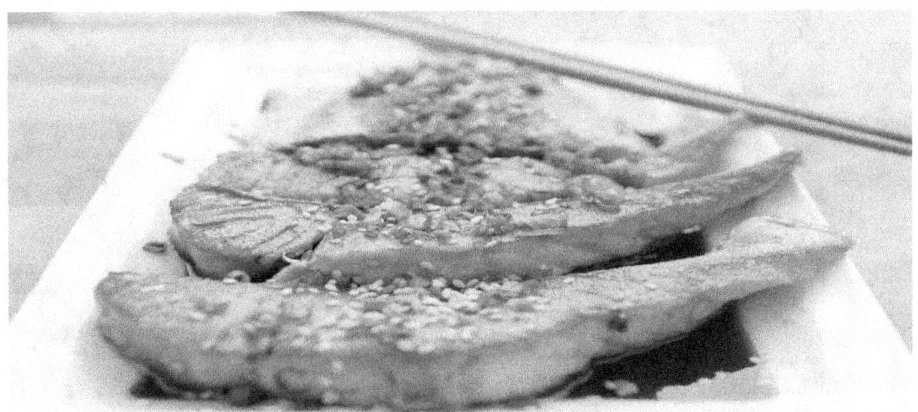

- **Identifying Foods with Ultra-Processing:** Understanding the distinguishing characteristics of ultra-processed foods — such as excessive quantities of added sugars, bad fats, salt, and artificial additives — helps participants identify these products. Individuals learn to become more discerning consumers by participating in label-reading activities and conversations. This helps individuals to discern ultra-processed products and choose healthier alternatives.

2) Development of Cooking Skills:

☐ **Practical Experience in Cooking:** Practical cooking workshops are a common component of food education programs, teaching students basic culinary skills, methods, and recipes utilizing whole, minimally processed products. Gaining self-assurance in the kitchen and learning how to make wholesome, straightforward meals from scratch gives people the capacity to take charge of their diets and lessen their need for highly processed foods.

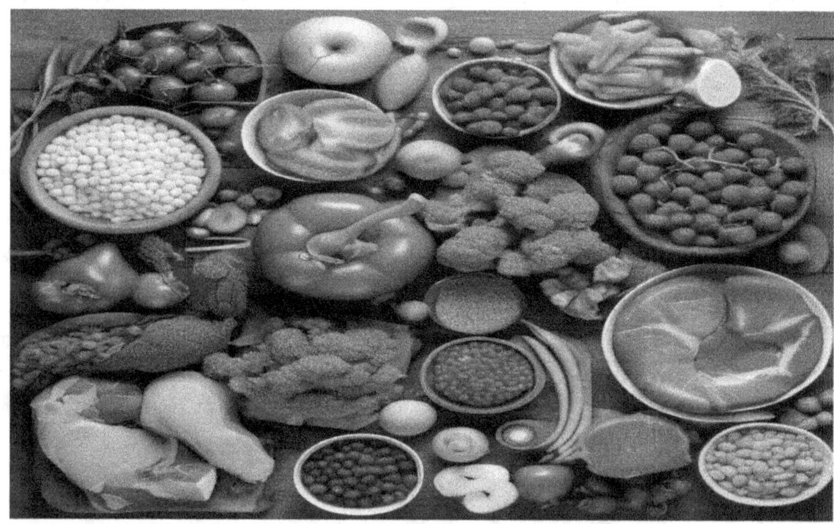

☐ **Encouraging Creative Culinary Practices:** Cooking lessons promote experimentation in the kitchen by encouraging participants to try different tastes, textures, and ingredients. People broaden their culinary horizons and learn new ways to appreciate whole foods by investigating other cuisines and cultural customs. This makes eating healthily more pleasurable and long-lasting in the long run.

3) Empowerment and Food Literacy:

- **Understanding Food Systems:** Participants in food education programs learn about the food system as a whole, including methods used in food production, processing, distribution, and marketing. People who have a deeper understanding of the intricacies of the food supply chain develop into more discerning consumers, capable of discerningly navigating product labels, marketing strategies, and industry influences.

- **Building Food Confidence:** Regardless of a person's socioeconomic status or level of culinary expertise, food literacy initiatives seek to increase their confidence and self-efficacy in choosing healthy food choices. These programs enable people to overcome obstacles to healthy eating and develop enduring eating habits that are consistent with their preferences and beliefs by offering helpful advice, tools, and support.

4) Community Engagement and Support:

- **Creating Supportive Environments:** Food education Initiatives encourage social support and community involvement by giving people a chance to interact with one another, connect with peers, and exchange experiences. These programs inspire group empowerment and resilience in adopting healthier lives by fostering a friendly atmosphere where participants may share ideas, recipes, and encouragement.

☐ **Addressing Food Insecurity**: Food education initiatives may help reduce food insecurity by giving people access to reasonable prices, wholesome foods, cooking supplies, and neighborhood-based support services. These initiatives aim to reduce food poverty and advance food sovereignty by giving people the knowledge and abilities to make the most of a few resources and guarantee that everyone has access to wholesome, culturally appropriate food.

5) Long-Term Health Benefits:

☐ **Preventing Diet-Related Diseases:** Food literacy and education programs have the potential to help prevent and lessen the effects of diet-related illnesses including diabetes, obesity, heart disease, and certain types of cancer. These initiatives enhance general health and well-being throughout the lifespan by supporting whole foods and reducing the consumption of ultra-processed meals rich in added sugars, harmful fats, and artificial additives.

☐ **Encouraging Sustainable Practices:** Food education programs provide a foundation of information about nutrition, culinary techniques, and food literacy that enables people to adopt long-lasting behavioral changes that promote long-term health and well-being. Whole foods, mindful eating, and enjoying food are prioritized by participants in their habits and routines, which results in long-lasting changes to their dietary habits and lifestyle choices.

Innovations in Food Production and Distribution as Solutions to Ultra-processed Foods

By using technology, sustainable practices, and customer preferences, food production, and distribution innovations provide viable alternatives for ultraprocessed meals by producing better, more nutrient-dense food choices. Let us examine in detail the following improvements in food production and distribution and their advantages over highly processed foods:

1) Sustainable Agriculture and Farming Methods:

☐ **Regenerative Agriculture:** Innovations in regenerative agriculture aim to restore soil health, enhance biodiversity, and trap carbon through holistic farming techniques like cover crops, crop rotation, and no-till farming. Regenerative agriculture provides nutrient-rich crops while reducing environmental damage and fostering long-term sustainability by placing a high priority on soil health and ecosystem resilience.

☐ **Vertical farming and Controlled environment agriculture:** Innovative technologies like hydroponics, aeroponics, and vertical stacking are used in vertical farming and controlled environment agriculture to grow fresh food inside year-round in regulated settings. Compared to conventional farming, these techniques use less land, water, and pesticides, which makes them more effective and sustainable for producing food in cities.

2) Other Sources of Protein:

☐ **Proteins Derived from Plants:** New developments in plant-based proteins, such as soy protein, lentil protein, and pea protein, provide sustainable substitutes for animal-based proteins with similar sensory qualities and nutritional value. The use of plant-based meat, dairy, and egg replacements is growing in favor among customers looking for more eco-friendly and healthful dietary choices.

- **Cell-Based Meat and Fish:** This technique eliminates the need for conventional animal husbandry by producing authentic animal meat and fish from cultivated animal cells. By using this novel strategy, it may be possible to lessen the negative environmental effects of the meat industry, enhance animal welfare, and solve issues with antibiotic resistance and food safety.

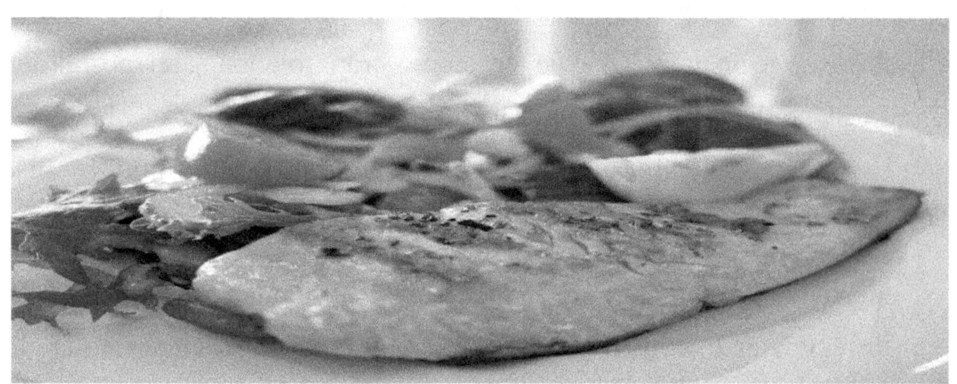

3) Functional Foods and Nutraceuticals:

- **Functional Ingredients:** To improve the nutritional value and health benefits of a broad variety of food and beverage products, functional ingredients including probiotics, prebiotics, fiber, antioxidants, and phytonutrients are included. Functional foods and nutraceuticals provide customers with easy and practical solutions to make dietary improvements by focusing on particular health issues including immune system support, gastrointestinal health, and cognitive performance.

☐ **Personalized Nutrition:** Customized dietary recommendations based on each person's genetic predispositions, metabolic profiles, and lifestyle characteristics are now possible due to advancements in personalized nutrition technologies, including microbiome analysis, DNA testing, and artificial intelligence algorithms. Consumers may maximize their nutritional intake and lower their risk of diet-related disorders by receiving personalized dietary guidance.

4) Direct-to-Consumer Distribution Models:

☐ **Online Grocery Platforms:** Online grocery platforms and direct-to-consumer delivery services allow consumers to access a vast range of fresh, local, and specialty foods from the comfort of their homes. These platforms enable consumers to buy whole foods, artisanal goods, and specialized ingredients without the need for conventional brick-and-mortar stores. They also provide convenience, transparency, and customization choices.

☐ **Community Supported Agriculture (CSA):** Through subscription-based business models, community-supported agriculture programs let consumers buy seasonal fruit, meats, dairy products, and other farm-fresh commodities directly from local farmers and producers. CSAs support small-scale farmers, advance sustainable agriculture, and improve community connections around food.

5) Food Waste Reduction and Circular Economy:

- **Upcycled Ingredients:** Technological advancements in this area turn food waste and byproducts from the food production process into wholesome components that can be added to food products. Fruit pomace, vegetable pulp, and wasted grains are examples of recycled materials that reduce food waste and increase resource efficiency in the food supply chain.

- **Circular Food Systems:** Circular food systems close the loop on food production, distribution, consumption, and disposal to reduce waste and increase resource efficiency. To produce value-added goods, restore soil health, and build a more resilient and sustainable food system, these systems place a high priority on techniques like composting, recycling, and repurposing food waste.

Advances in food production and distribution, which combine technology, sustainable practices, and consumer desires to provide healthier, more nutrient-dense food choices, present viable substitutes and answers to ultra-processed meals.

Chapter 9

Case Studies and Success Stories

Communities and Countries Taking Action Against Ultra-processed Foods

Around the globe, nations and communities are proactively addressing the problems posed by ultra-processed foods and encouraging their citizens to adopt healthy eating habits. These efforts have reduced the use of ultra-processed foods, improved nutritional outcomes, and improved general well-being via a mix of governmental measures, education initiatives, community collaborations, and public health campaigns. Let's look at some case studies and achievements of nations and communities that have fought against highly processed foods:

1) Brazil:

☐ **The Brazilian Dietary Guidelines:** Brazil's dietary guidelines updated in 2014 place a strong emphasis on eating fresh, locally produced, minimally processed foods while avoiding ultra-processed items that are rich in harmful fats, added sugars, and salt. These recommendations provide a thorough framework for encouraging better eating practices and directing the creation of national policy.

☐ **Food Labeling Regulations:** Brazil has imposed front-of-package labeling laws that mandate the use of warning warnings on packaged goods that are

excessive in salt, unhealthy fats, and added sugars. These labels assist customers in making educated decisions and lower consumption of highly processed goods. They include a red warning flag and clear wording indicating excessive sugar, fat, or salt levels.

2) Mexico:

☐ **Tax on Sugar-Sweetened Beverages:** In 2014, Mexico imposed a national tax on sugar-sweetened drinks to address the growing prevalence of obesity and diabetes. The tax, which is levied on sugar-filled drinks, has been effective in lowering consumption and raising money for public health programs that encourage healthy lives and lower the incidence of illnesses linked to food.

☐ **Active Living and Healthy Eating Initiative:** The Healthy Eating and Active Living Initiative (HEAL) in Mexico is a broad public health initiative designed to lower childhood and adolescent obesity rates, encourage better eating habits, and increase physical activity. HEAL consists of legislative efforts, community-based interventions, and educational programs aimed at communities, workplaces, and schools.

3) Japan:

☐ **Shokuiku (Food Education) Program:** Shokuiku is a nationwide program in Japan that aims to prevent diet-related illnesses and encourage better eating habits via culinary skills training and food education. The program places a strong focus on the cultural value of traditional Japanese food, which is distinguished by its use of fresh, seasonal ingredients, balanced flavors, and elegant presentation.

- **Farm-to-School Programs:** In Japan, there is a collaboration between local farmers and schools to prepare fresh, locally sourced ingredients for school meals. School menus including traditional Japanese foods and seasonal vegetables encourage kids to make better eating choices, support local farmers, and teach them the value of sustainable and high-quality food.

4) United States:

- **The Healthy, Hunger-Free Kids Act:** The Healthy, Hunger-Free Kids Act of 2010 significantly changed the National School Lunch Program and School Breakfast Program in the United States. These changes included updated school meal nutrition guidelines, easier access to fruits, vegetables, and whole grains, and limitations on the sale of competing foods that are rich in fat, sugar, and sodium.

Community-Based Initiatives: Innovative projects and programs are being implemented in American communities all around the country to encourage better eating settings and lower consumption of highly processed foods. Instances include communal gardens, farmers' markets, health-conscious corner store endeavors, and urban agriculture programs that augment the availability of wholesome, fresh produce in marginalized areas.

5) European Union:

- **European Strategy aims to prevent Non-Communicable Diseases (NCDs) via interventions:** Obesity, diabetes, and cardiovascular disease are among the non-communicable illnesses for which the European Union has established a comprehensive preventative plan. To assist customers make educated decisions, this approach calls for actions to enhance food labeling, restrict the marketing of harmful foods to youngsters, and encourage the consumption of healthy diets.

- ☐ **Package Front Labeling:** Front-of-package labeling systems have been introduced in some European nations to assist consumers in making better food choices and cutting down on the intake of ultra-processed foods. These labeling methods make it simpler for consumers to quickly make better decisions by using color-coded labels or symbols to show the nutritional quality of packaged items.

In conclusion, nations and communities everywhere are proactively tackling the problems posed by highly processed foods and encouraging their citizens to adopt healthy eating habits.

Corporate Initiatives and Responsibility in Addressing Ultra-processed Foods

Corporate initiatives and responsibility are essential in tackling the problems related to ultra-processed foods. Now let's examine corporate responsibility and efforts in more detail using case studies and success stories:

1) Nestlé:

- ☐ **Nutritional Reformulation:** One of the largest food and beverage companies in the world - Nestlé, has been working to reformulate its products to lower the amount of salt, harmful fats, and added sugars. Nestlé wants to help people make better food choices and lessen the negative effects of ultra-processed meals on public health. To do this, it is working to improve the nutritional profile of its products and provide healthier alternatives.

☐ **Portion Control and Marketing Strategies:** With a focus on children, Nestlé has launched campaigns to encourage portion management and ethical marketing techniques. Nestlé aims to promote moderation and balanced eating habits among consumers, particularly in vulnerable groups, by providing smaller portion sizes and restricting the promotion of harmful items to youngsters.

2) Danone:

☐ **Health and Sustainability as Priorities**: The global food products company Danone has made sustainability and health a priority in all aspects of its business operations. Danone is dedicated to encouraging wholesome, sustainable food choices and minimizing the environmental effects of its operations and products. Examples of these programs include the Danone Ecosystem Fund and One Planet. One Health platform.

☐ **Collaborations for Effect:** Danone works in partnership with a range of stakeholders, such as governments, non-governmental organizations, and educational institutions, to tackle urgent issues concerning ultra-processed foods and public health. Danone wants to build a more sustainable and healthy future for everyone by promoting positive change in the food system via partnerships and group action.

3) Unilever:

☐ **The Unilever Sustainable Living Plan:** Unilever has introduced the Unilever Sustainable Living Plan, a comprehensive strategy aimed at enhancing the global health and well-being of people globally while diminishing the ecological impact of its products and operations. Also, through programs like the "Health & Well-Being" pillar, Unilever aims to decrease the amount of fat, sugar, and salt in its products, promote nutrition labeling, and encourage better and healthier diets.

- ☐ **Empowering Consumers:** Unilever is dedicated to providing consumers with the information and resources they need to choose healthier foods. Unilever empowers people to make knowledgeable choices about their food purchases and dietary practices by offering clear, science-based information via educational campaigns, nutrition labeling initiatives, and digital platforms.

4) Whole Foods Market:

- ☐ **Commitment to Whole Foods:** Whole Foods Market, One of the top retailers of natural and organic goods, places a high value on whole, minimally processed foods in both its product selection and marketing campaigns. A whole meal Market encourages consumers to prioritize nutrient-rich meals over ultra-processed ones by providing a wide variety of fresh vegetables, whole grains, lean meats, and natural ingredients. This helps consumers make better dietary choices.

- ☐ **Education and Transparency:** Whole Foods Market is committed to educating consumers and being open and honest about the origin, manufacturing process, and nutritional value of their products. Through initiatives like Whole Foods Market, Health Starts Here, and in-store labeling systems, the retailer enables customers to make knowledgeable choices about their food purchases and eating patterns.

5) Patagonia Provisions:

☐ **Sustainable Food Products:** The food branch of an outdoor apparel company called Patagonia Provisions is dedicated to creating sustainably sourced food items that prioritize social responsibility, health, and environmental stewardship. With products ranging from organic grains and beans to wild-caught seafood and regeneratively sourced meats. Patagonia Provisions provides wholesome, ethically produced alternatives to ultra-processed goods.

☐ **Regenerative Agriculture Initiatives:** Patagonia Provisions collaborates with farmers, ranchers, and conservation groups to promote regenerative agriculture practices that improve soil health, increase biodiversity, and sequester carbon. Patagonia Provisions seeks to solve the underlying causes of food system challenges and create a positive environmental and social impact by endorsing regenerative agricultural projects.

Chapter 10

Future Perspectives and Recommendations

Long-term Health Projections

Long-term health predictions provide important information about how dietary habits, such as consuming a lot of ultra-processed food, may affect population health over time. Now, let's examine long-term health estimates in detail and provide some suggestions and future views.

1) The Burden of disease and epidemiological trends:

- **Rising Rates of Diet-Related Diseases:** Long-term health projections show that the prevalence of diet-related diseases, including obesity, diabetes, cardiovascular disease, and some cancers, will be on the increase. This trend is being driven by factors like ultra-processed food consumption, sedentary lifestyles, and unhealthy eating habits. These illnesses put a heavy strain on healthcare systems and raise the risk of early death, worse quality of life, and higher healthcare costs.

- **Health Disparities and Inequities:** Long-term forecasts also show disparities in health outcomes across socioeconomic groupings, racial and ethnic populations, and geographic areas, with disadvantaged people disproportionately impacted by poor nutrition and diet-related illnesses. Health inequalities can be addressed through targeted interventions that

address socioeconomic determinants of health, advance food justice, and guarantee that everyone has access to good, healthy affordable food alternatives.

2) Policy Implications and Public Health Interventions:

☐ **Regulatory Measures:** Healthy eating habits, restriction of exposure to harmful ingredients, and reduction of ultra-processed food consumption are all urgently needed, as long-term health forecasts make clear to promote the population level. Also, Restrictions on marketing, sugar taxes, food labeling laws, and subsidies for nutritious foods are a few examples of policies that might help foster a culture of health and lower the incidence of diet-related illnesses.

☐ **Nutrition Education Programs:** Funding public health campaigns and nutrition education programs is crucial to educating people about the negative health effects of ultra-processed foods and enabling them to make educated food choices. These programs need to focus on a variety of demographics and include tools for encouraging healthy eating habits from infancy through maturity, as well as instruction in culinary skills and culturally appropriate messages.

3) Innovative Solutions and Technological Advancement:

☐ **Food Innovation and Reformulation:** The development of healthier, more nutritious substitutes for ultra-processed foods may result in diverse food innovations in the food industry. Policymakers may encourage a move toward better food alternatives that support long-term health by providing incentives to companies to decrease the amounts of harmful fats, added sugars, and salt in their products and increase the inclusion of whole, minimally processed components.

☐ **Technology and Digital Health Solutions:** Wearables, telehealth platforms, and mobile applications are examples of digital health solutions that can be used to support healthy lifestyle choices, encourage adherence to eating habits, and help people change their behavior. These technologies enable people to take charge of their health and well-being by offering social support networks, real-time feedback, and individualized dietary guidance.

4) Environmental Aspects of Sustainable Food Systems:

☐ **Encouraging Sustainable Diets:** Long-term health projections highlight how crucial it is to encourage sustainable diets that not only support human health but also reduce their negative effects on the environment as well as advance global health. Plant-based diets and other sustainable eating practices lessen the need for animal products, cut down on greenhouse gas emissions, protect natural resources, and encourage biodiversity preservation—all of which help to create a food system that is more robust and sustainable for future generations.

☐ **Addressing Food Waste:** Long-term health projections highlight the need to address food waste and supply chain inefficiencies since these factors lead to resource depletion, environmental degradation, and economic losses. A more sustainable and reasonable food system may be achieved by implementing strategies to reduce food waste, such as better distribution and storage systems, consumer education initiatives, and laws requiring the redistribution of excess food to those in need.

Ultra-processed foods.......

Conclusion

Processed foods are foods that have been changed from their original condition in some manner, such as by the addition of preservatives, the removal of particular constituents, or the use of processing procedures like freezing or canning. Processed foods may include a broad variety of goods, such as canned vegetables, frozen meals, and snack foods like chips or cookies.

There is continuous discussion concerning the possible health implications of processed foods. Some studies show that a diet heavy in processed foods may raise the risk of certain health disorders. Other study shows that certain processed foods may give some health advantages, such as convenience and enhanced availability of certain nutrients.

It is essential to highlight that not all processed foods are bad, and there are various methods to include them in a balanced diet. The idea is to pick processed meals that are nutrient-dense and created with whole ingredients and to minimize the quantity of highly processed foods. It is also a good idea to balance processed meals with a range of healthy, less processed foods including fruits, vegetables, and whole grains.

It is crucial to highlight that although ultra-processed meals might have detrimental short-term health impacts, these effects can be minimized by having a balanced diet that includes a range of complete, unprocessed

foods. It is also crucial to be cautious of portion sizes and to participate in regular physical exercise <u>to</u> maintain a healthy weight and general health.